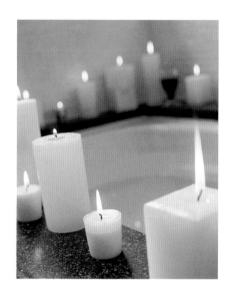

# detox

### for life

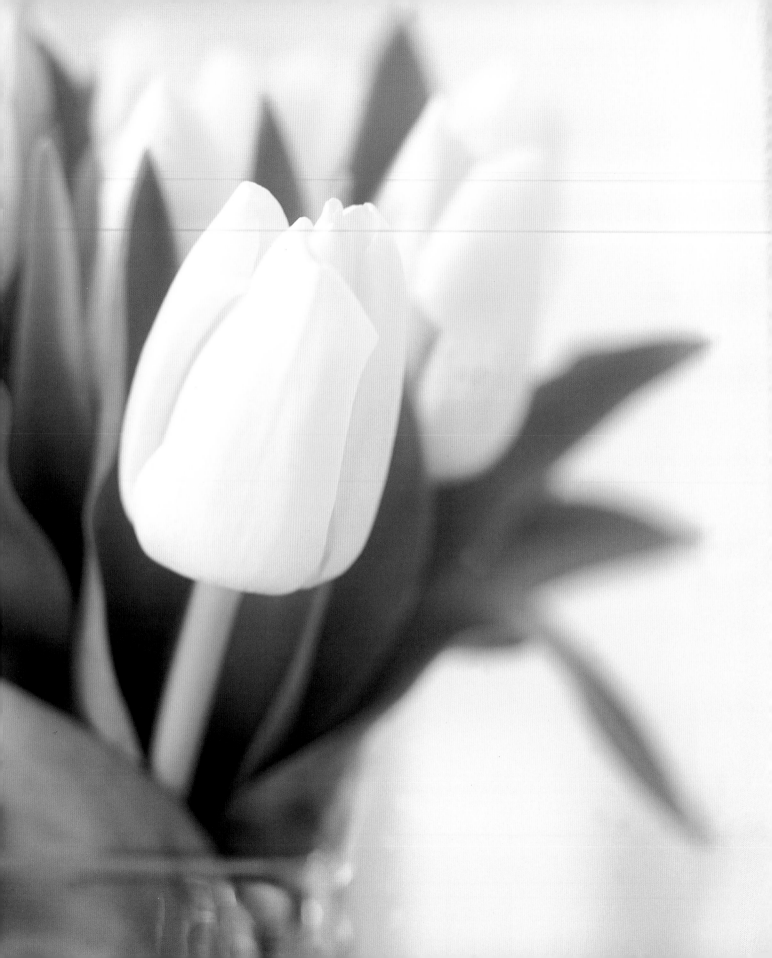

# detox
## for life

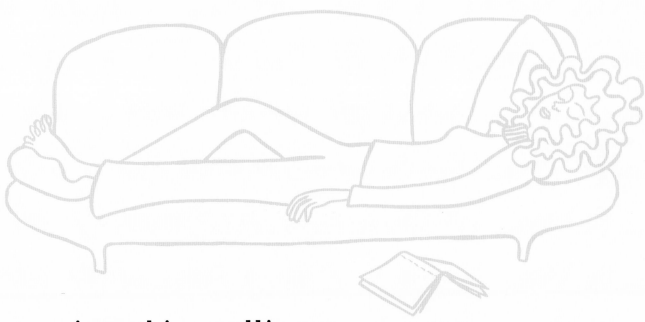

josephine collins

with photography by polly wreford

RYLAND
PETERS
& SMALL
LONDON NEW YORK

**Illustrations** Olga Rezontova
**Editorial consultant** Christina Rodenbeck
**Nutritional advisor** Penny Crowther

First published in the USA in 2003
This paperback edition published in 2006 by
Ryland Peters & Small, Inc.
519 Broadway
5th Floor
New York, NY 10012
www.rylandpeters.com
10 9 8 7 6 5 4 3 2 1

ISBN-10: 1 84597 091 8
ISBN-13: 978 1 84597 091 8

**Library of Congress Cataloging-in-Publication Data**
*The original edition of this book was cataloged as follows:*
Collins, Josephine.
  Detox for life: purify your mind, body, and soul/ Josephine Collins;
with photography by Polly Wreford.
    p. cm.
Includes index.
  ISBN 1-84172-486-6
  1. Detoxification (Health)  I. Title.
  RA784.5.C66 2003
  613—dc21
                                        2003006726

Printed and bound in China.

Neither the author nor the publisher can be held
responsible for any claim arising out of the use or
misuse of suggestions made in this book. While every
effort has been made to ensure that the information
contained in the book is accurate and up to date, it is
advisory only and should not be used as an alternative
to seeking specialized medical advice. Anyone suffering
from a medical condition or an allergy should consult
a doctor before starting a detox program, and detox
programs should be avoided altogether in pregnancy.

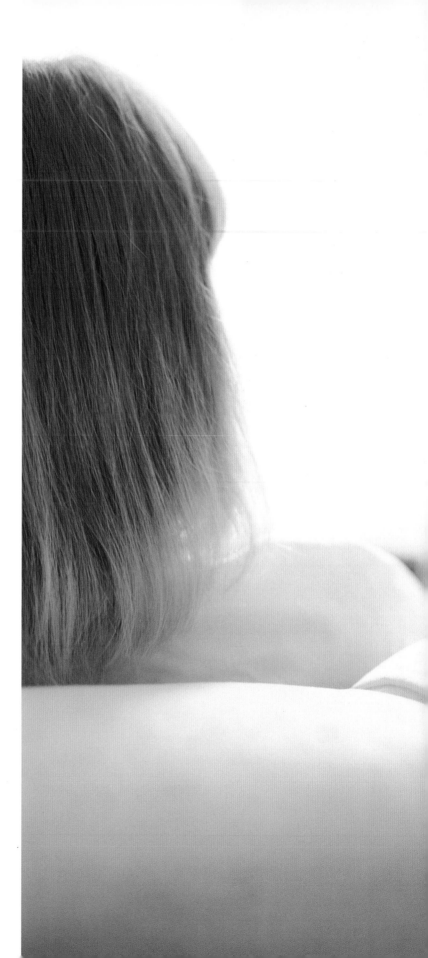

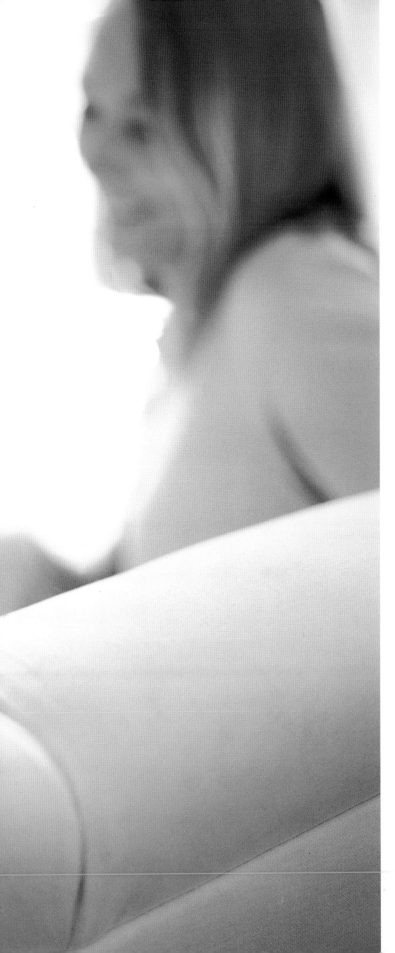

# contents

introduction     6

## detox your mind     8
step 1   know what you want     12
step 2   make a plan     14
step 3   do the energy work     20
step 4   take action     26
step 5   let go of worries     30
do it now     32

## detox your body     34
step 1   eat well     38
step 2   exercise effectively     48
step 3   enjoy your sleep     52
step 4   purify from the outside     54
step 5   use the power tools     60
do it now     66

## detox your relationships     68
step 1   know who you are     72
step 2   know how you are seen     78
step 3   value people     82
step 4   empower youself     90
do it now     94

## detox your space     96
step 1   what your home says     100
step 2   know what comes in     104
step 3   clear that clutter     106
step 4   create an energy flow     110
step 5   cleanse and refresh     118
do it now     120

final word     122
picture credits     127
index     128

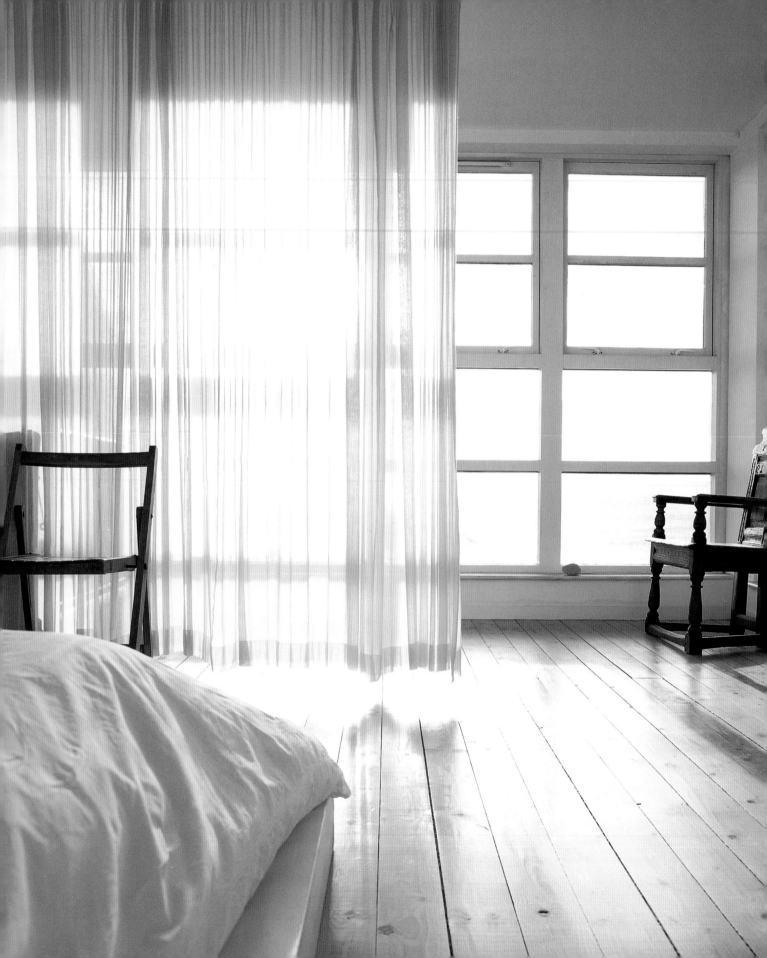

# introduction

The fast pace of modern life can leave us feeling physically, emotionally, and mentally overwhelmed and overloaded. We get caught up on a daily treadmill that absorbs so much of our time and energy that we never manage to fulfill our true potential. We perform a skillful juggling act to satisfy the demands of career, running a home, sharing a love life, bringing up a family, balancing household finances, and staying healthy. Add to these the information explosion, the benefits of new technology, and the temptations of consumerism—and it is hardly surprising that many of us become so distracted that we lose track of who we really are and what we really want.

*Detox for Life* is about stepping off that treadmill and taking the time to start creating the life you really want to live. It is about learning to accentuate the positive and transforming or letting go of those things that stop you from being happy and fulfilled—whether this is an unhealthy relationship, a bad diet, or negative thinking.

It is my belief that, to find genuine fulfillment, we should look at our lives holistically. It's no good having a perfect body and feeling depressed, or having a beautiful home that is too untidy to appreciate. How we manage one area of our life has a knock-on effect on other areas, so to create true harmony and balance, you should aim to have all the elements of your life working well. That's why this book tackles mind, body, relationships, and space—four essential areas where you can make immediate and positive changes that will bring about a real difference. My aim is to provide you with the tools to do just that.

The book is designed so that you can either read and work through it from cover to cover or pick an area that's important to you and concentrate on that first—so start wherever you like. I have created a series of step-by-step plans to help you move easily through each chapter. As you work through the book, you should notice your life becoming better organized and more focused, freeing you to do those things you really enjoy. By pacing yourself well and tackling each problem gradually, you will find that your life has improved beyond measure.

Detoxing is a continuing process and this book should help you initiate the changes you need to improve the quality of your life. Even when you have completed the whole program, you may want to come back to it periodically to refresh and boost certain areas. The transition into health, harmony, and balance should be a positive one, so I hope you will come to treasure *Detox for Life* and regard it as a supportive and inspiring friend.

Josephine Collins

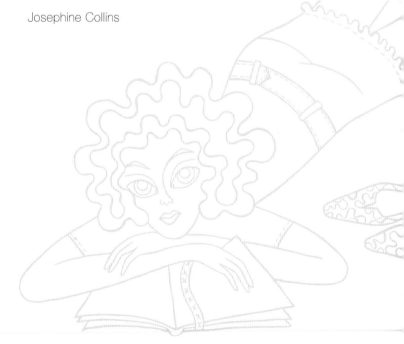

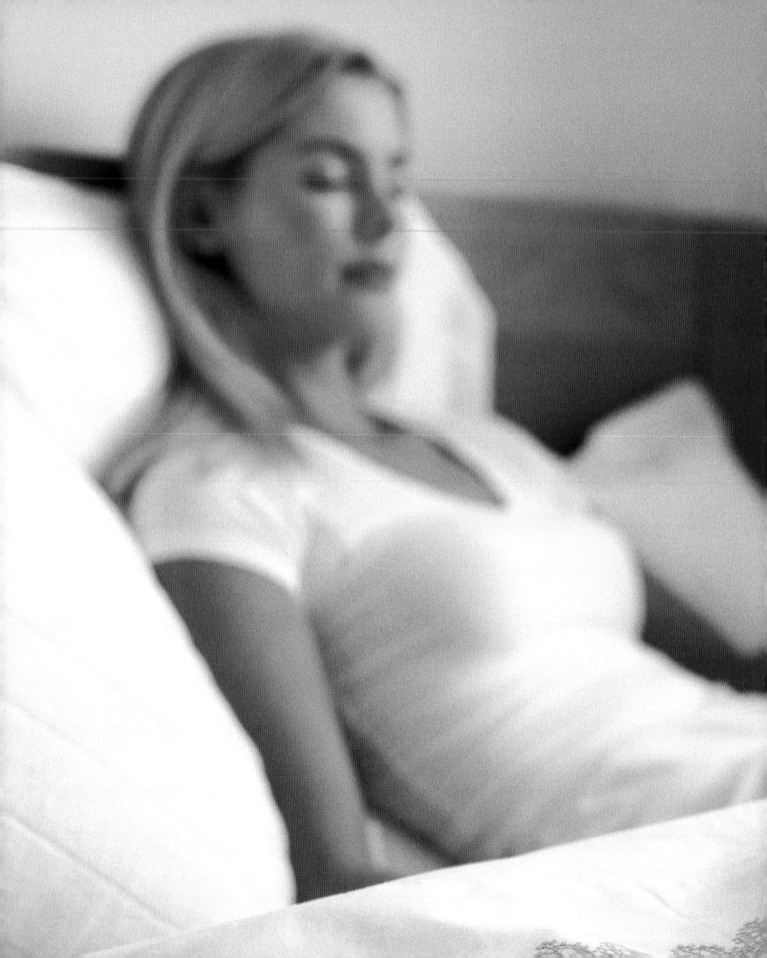

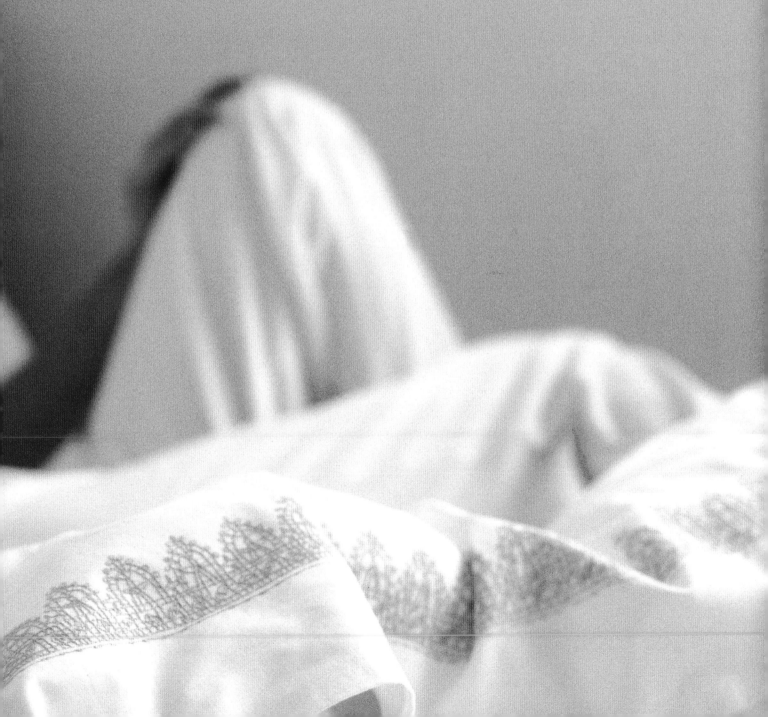

detox
your mind

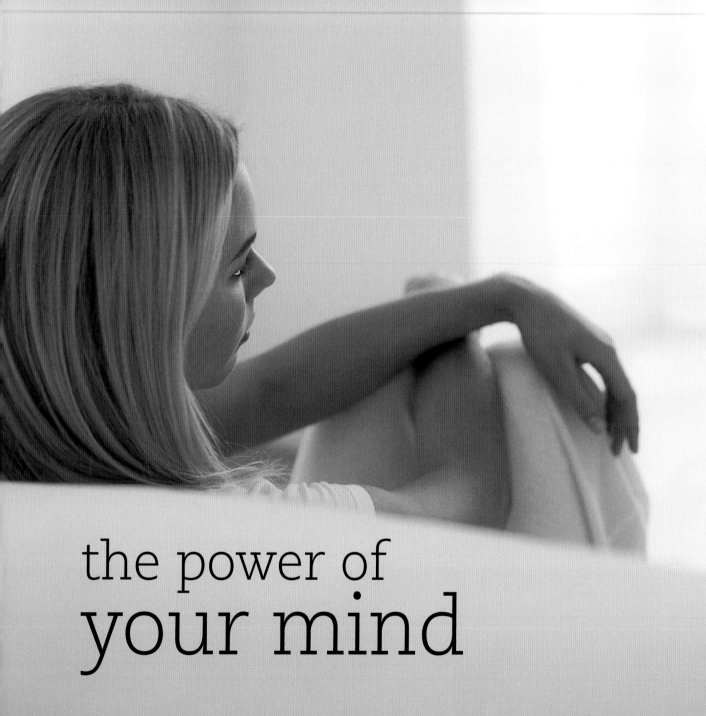

# the power of
# your mind

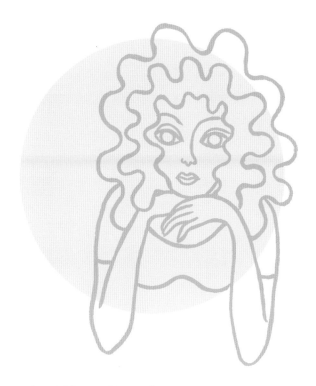

Your mind is one of your most powerful assets. When it works well, you can think rationally, make clear decisions, and pursue your goals with confidence. But with the myriad distractions of modern life it is easy for your mental processes to become overworked and overloaded, leading to confusion, stress, and negative thinking.

This chapter focuses on being clear about what you want to achieve and provides you with the tools for laying down an effective plan of action that will help you find true fulfillment. One aim is to get your mind working for you instead of against you, so the skills of visualization and self-talk are fully explained.

By completing the five steps to detoxing your mind described on the following pages, you will benefit from a mental workout that will give you an opportunity to rethink your goals and reassess your priorities.

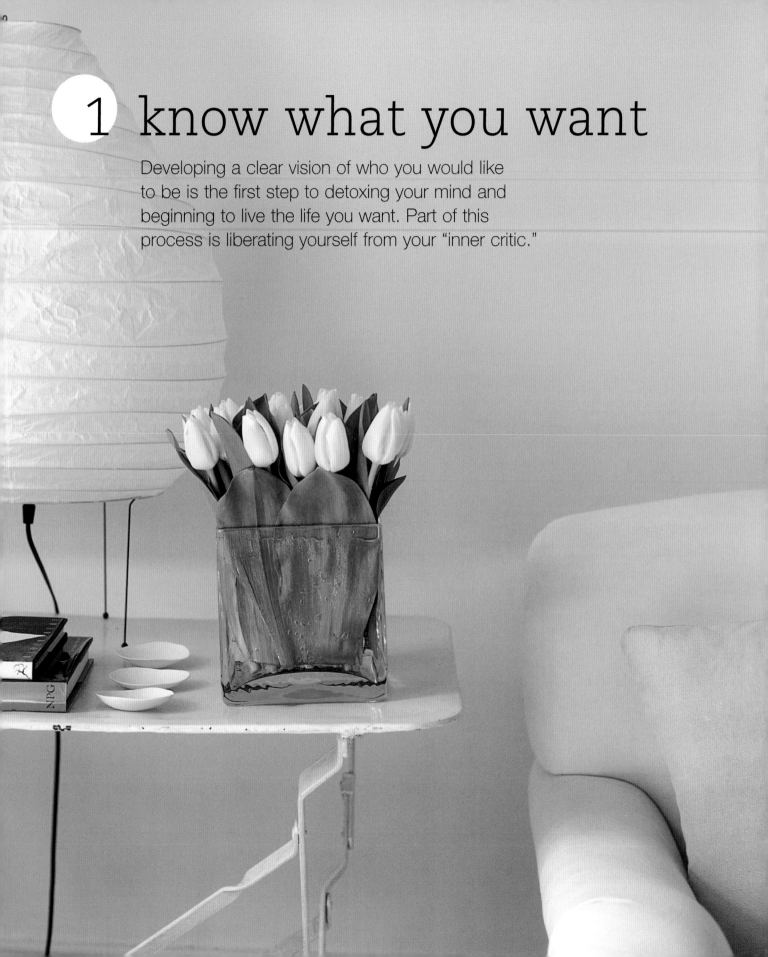

# 1 know what you want

Developing a clear vision of who you would like
to be is the first step to detoxing your mind and
beginning to live the life you want. Part of this
process is liberating yourself from your "inner critic."

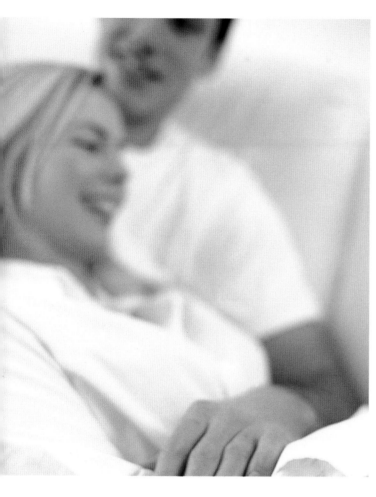

If you really want to make a better life for yourself, you need a vision that you can commit to. So, if there is something in your vision of yourself and your life that you really don't believe in, let it go. It is pointless holding up an ideal that you are not willing or able to work toward. Unrealistic goals are always disheartening and will give you a sense of failure before you have even begun.

If, on the other hand, you have a vision that is out of reach at this moment but that you believe is achievable, even if you don't know how, let this be your goal. Don't be afraid to think big. You only live once, so go for your dreams and get what you want out of life.

## handling your inner critic

Most people have an inner critic in their head that pipes up every now and again, telling them that they can't do something, that they don't deserve it, or that they are not good enough.

Although your inner critic may seem to be a negative force, it does not always work against you. Sometimes it may be attempting to keep your behavior in check or trying to protect you from making a mistake. But its views may not always be up to date. It could be acting in accordance with habits acquired in childhood or in response to comments made by other people. Your inner critic's intervention in some situations may not be relevant any more and could be getting in the way of your good intentions.

If this is the case, your inner critic must be kept in check. When you hear the voice in your head saying that you can't do something or that you lack the necessary qualities, say silently to yourself "Stop!" and replace the message with a positive statement. For example, if you are in an interview and hear your inner critic murmuring, "I'm too nervous, I won't get the job," say "Stop!" and replace the criticism with a statement such as: "I am calm and confident. I can handle this interview easily."

If you keep doing this every time your critic comes up with a negative statement that doesn't serve your purpose, you will find that your thought habits gradually become more positive and your inner critic loses the power to sabotage your efforts.

## your personal vision

Fulfillment, like success, carries different meanings for different people. What does it mean to you? Set aside a few minutes to shut your eyes and imagine the person you would like to be and the life you desire. Would you like to be more attractive or richer? Would you like to have a better job? If you had your ideal life, would you be more confident, feel more in control? Would your life be more organized? Would you have a different partner?

When you have finished thinking about your ideal self, write down a description of your vision. Is there any reason why you can't turn yourself into the person you want to be and create the lifestyle you seek? If the answer is yes, is the reason valid—or does the blame lie with your inner critic, that small voice in your head that so often holds you back?

# 2 make a plan

If you examine your life objectively, the areas that need detoxing will become clearer, enabling you to devise a plan. It is time to start making your vision of the future a reality.

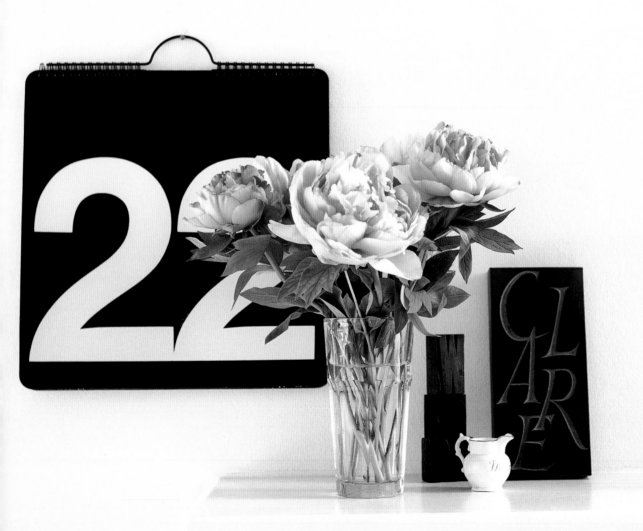

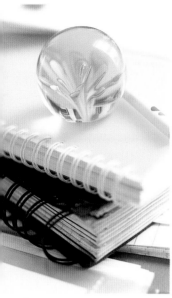

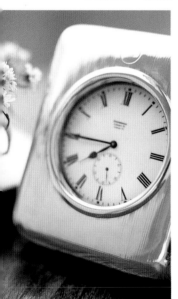

### transforming your vision into reality

Start by deciding where you need to focus time and energy. On a legal pad write the following headings, leaving plenty of space between each: Health, Money, Relationships, Family, Career, Social Life, Possessions, Other. (Other covers anything else that is important to you, such as spiritual practices, learning, pampering yourself, and hobbies.)

Under each heading, write down everything relating to that specific area that you would like to have, to do, or to be. Then review the lists and ask yourself the following questions about each goal you have included:

*Am I willing to put in the physical, mental, and emotional work needed to achieve this goal?*

*Am I willing to make a plan of action and follow it through to achieve this goal?*

*Does this goal contradict or cancel out any of the other goals on my list?*

*Will this goal take me toward my vision?*

In response to how well each goal stands up to close scrutiny, you can leave it alone, adjust it, or cross it off the list. Then give each surviving goal one, two, or three checks according to how important and urgent it seems to you—three being the most important.

Count up how many goals you have marked with three checks, how many with two, and how many with one. If you count at least ten goals that have either three or two checks, set aside those that have only one. You can always tackle the leftover goals later.

Keep eliminating goals from your list until you have just ten left. Then, on a new sheet of paper, write down the ten goals in the order of their importance.

Next to each goal, write down how you will know when you have achieved it. Be as specific as you can. For example, if one of your goals is to be rich, what does this mean to you? Does it mean $10 million in the bank, a mansion in the country, or something else? When you are clear in your own mind about the results, you will know when to cross each goal off your list.

make a list of
all the things
you would
like to have,
to do, or to be

### setting priorities

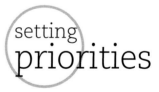

✓ = I want to achieve this goal

✓✓ = this goal is important and I want to achieve it

✓✓✓ = this goal is very important and I really want to achieve it

# where to go from here

Review your goals, then decide which of the statements below applies to you and refer to the relevant section of the book.

It would it be easier to achieve my goals if:

- I had more confidence
- I conquered my fears
- I had more time

continue reading this section, *detox your mind* (pages 8–33).

- I looked better
- I lost weight
- I had more energy

see *detox your body* (pages 34–67).

- I understood myself better
- I understood others better
- I transformed or let go of a current relationship or friendship

see *detox your relationships* (pages 68–95).

- I was better organized
- I had a more attractive home
- I had more money

see *detox your space* (pages 96–125).

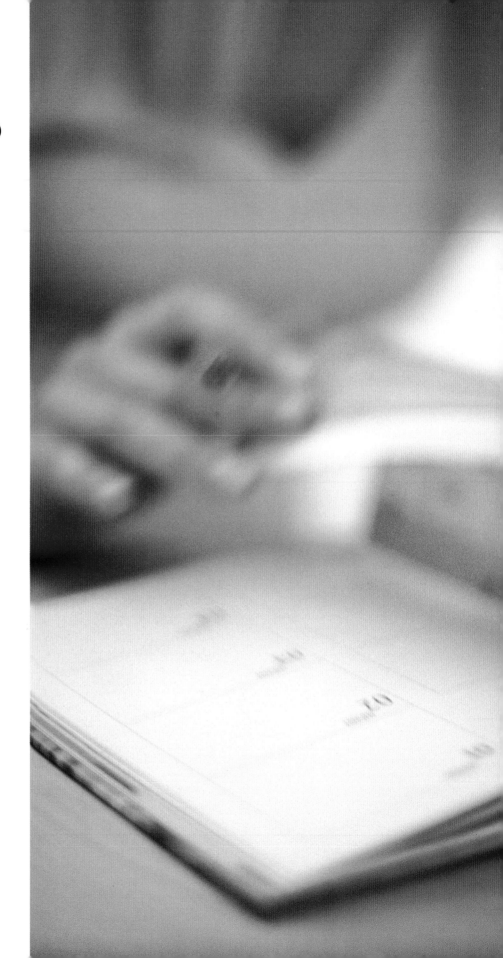

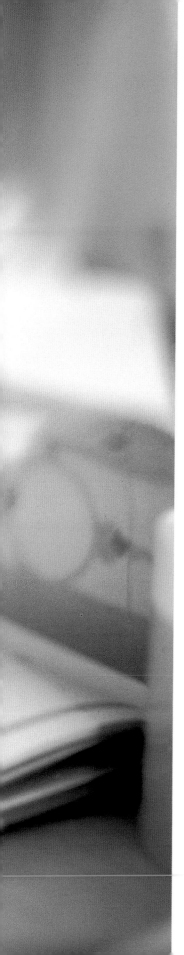
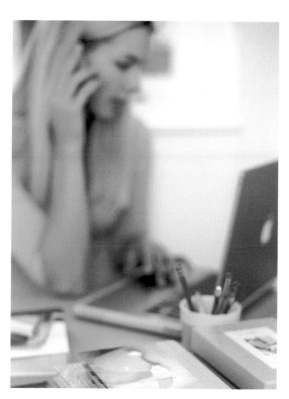

## making room for success

Now that you have your top ten goals to concentrate on, it is time to work out how you can detox your life and free up the time, energy, and space needed to achieve them.

Start by looking at the statements listed on the opposite page and establish which section of the book focuses on resolving the issues and concerns that are particularly relevant to you. You can then decide which section you would like to work on first.

One way to determine the order in which you want to detox your life is to think about which area, once detoxed, will liberate the most time, energy, or space for you. You could concentrate on the area that will help you realize your goals faster—or you could work on the area that seems likely to prove the easiest or the most difficult to detox.

The next move is to devise a plan of action. Life is too short to wait until you've cleared out what you don't want in order to make way for what you do. So your top ten goals and your detox plan should work hand in hand. For example, if one of your most important goals is to have a slim, healthy figure, one of your detox tasks might be to clear out your refrigerator and fill it with healthy food and drink.

Now that you have formulated both your goals and your detox priorities, you need to break them down into achievable steps within an allotted time frame—so have your diary ready.

## figuring out how to achieve your goals

Take a new piece of paper and on the left-hand side write down the top ten goals that you arrived at by doing the exercise on page 15, leaving plenty of space between each. Then next to each goal write down the steps you think will be required to accomplish each goal and the time scale needed. Could it be done in a week or a month, or might it take as long as a year? It will of course be guesswork, but try to choose a reasonable completion date for each goal.

Once you have a clear idea of the time frame you are working within, you can divide up the steps and write them down in the relevant place in your diary, ready to be ticked off as they are accomplished. For example, you may want to learn a new language. You could decide to put aside one hour a day or one day a week for focused study. While you don't want to move the goal posts too often, it makes sense to be flexible. Life is a dynamic process, and goals and priorities can shift. You may also find that your ideas and desires change as you move closer to realizing your aims, so be willing to update and adapt your program when necessary.

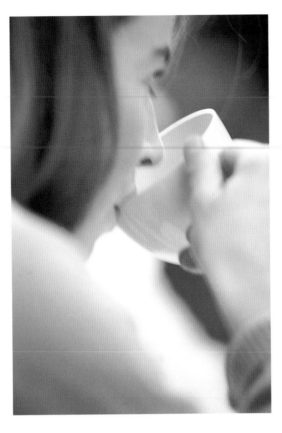

### planning your detox

Now that you have specified your goals and worked out a strategy to achieve them, you need to devise a detox program.

When you first embark on a detox regime, you will have to set aside substantial periods of time to sort out and resolve those aspects of your life that need special attention. This is especially crucial in the case of areas that have been neglected for a long while. For this reason, the best times to devote to your detox tasks are likely to be weekends or evenings. So consult your calendar and allocate the length of time you think will

be necessary to focus on each element of your detox. It may take a weekend to clear out your closet, or you may want to set aside an evening to talk over an important issue with a friend. You could decide to allocate one hour of every evening for a week to filing your papers, or one weekend at the end of the month to focus on detoxing your body.

The speed at which you work through your detox is up to you. Since you may not know what tasks lie ahead until you reach the relevant section of the book, and you don't always know how long a task will take, a bit of guesswork is needed. But the very process of going through your diary and setting aside time to detox your life shows that you have made a commitment to yourself—and forward planning makes it harder to use the excuse that you can't fit your detoxing tasks into your hectic schedule.

When you are working through the chapters that follow, you may find that some of the detox tasks are already incorporated into the steps you have set out to reach your goals—which can only be a bonus.

Initially, it may seem that the combination of following a detox plan and working to realize your goals leaves you with less time than you started with. However, once the main detox tasks have been accomplished and you have implemented a detox plan of action to keep your days free from the things that drain you, you should find that you have far more time, energy, and space than before—and a more successful life to go with it.

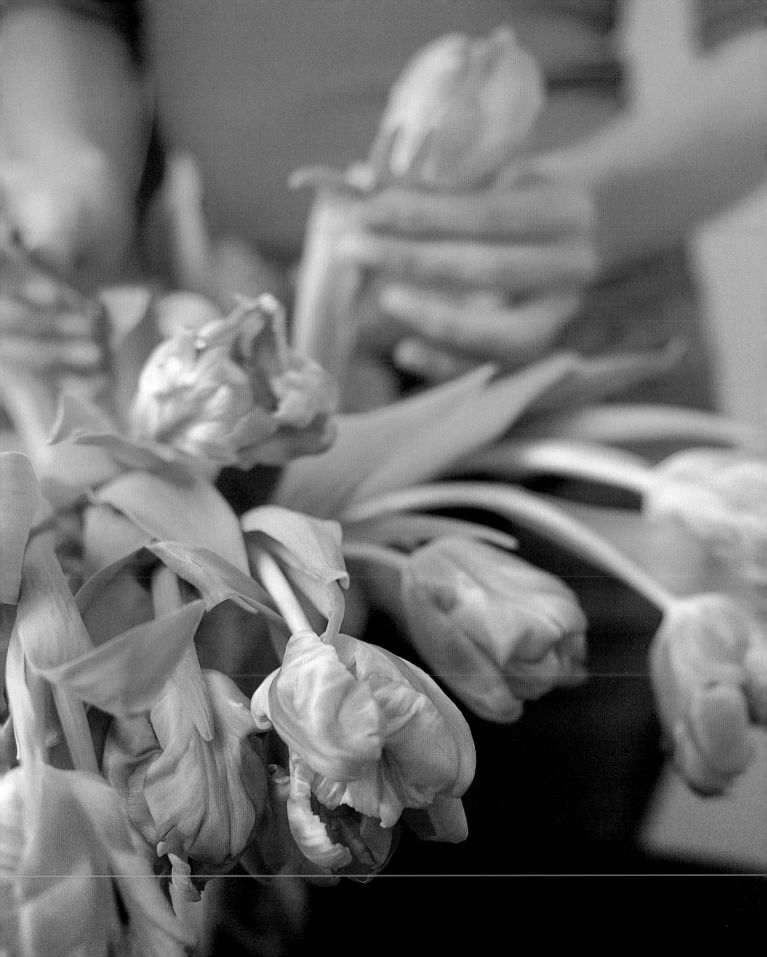

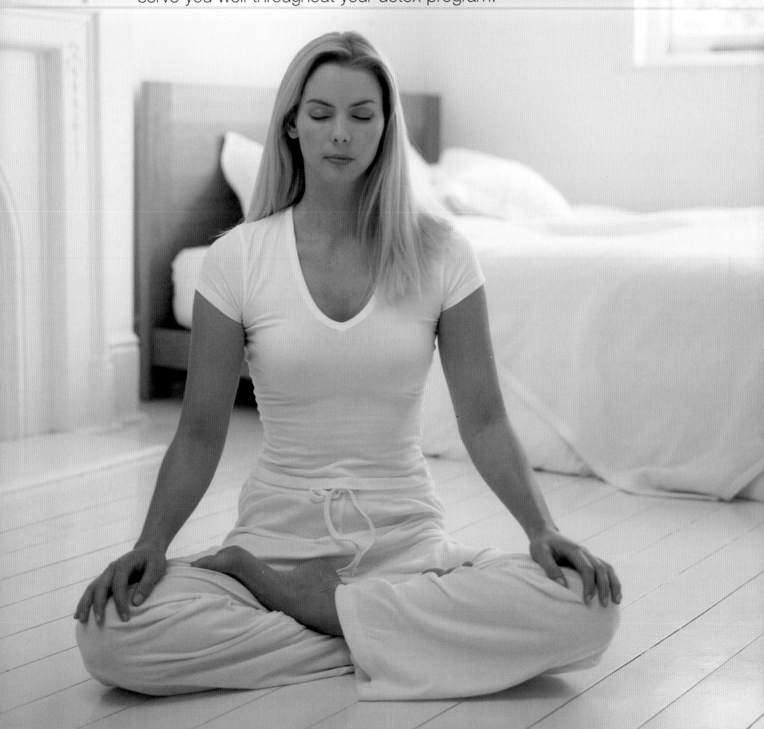

# 3 do the energy work

Learn techniques that help you to increase your inner resolve and your sense of personal power. These will serve you well throughout your detox program.

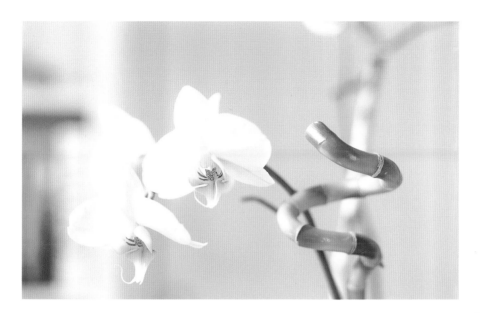

the conscious mind can reinforce the subconscious to produce strong results

## paving the way to success

No one entirely understands how the mind works or how powerful it is, but the general belief is that it is divided into two parts: the conscious and the subconscious. The conscious mind, which we are aware of, is responsible for the practical, logical side of thoughts and actions. The subconscious mind controls physical functions such as breathing and circulation, and is responsible for dreaming, intuition, and creativity.

Just as you use your conscious mind to make plans and take actions, you can use your subconscious to build self-esteem and bring inspiration and insight. Two ways of doing this are through visualization and self-talk.

Your subconscious is especially receptive to symbols or pictures and also to words you say to yourself. For this reason, using your imagination to affirm what you want can be a powerful tool in achieving your goals. The conscious and subconscious complement each other, and used together, they can bring impressive results.

## the art of visualization

Part of detoxing your mind is being clear about what you want, and visualization is a powerful technique for getting your subconcious mind to work with you toward your goals. You often use the visualization process when you think and make decisions, and you also use it at night while you dream and when you are doing something artistic. Visualization is just another way to describe your imagination and its ability to create pictures in the mind.

Some people find conscious visualization techniques easy to master; others find them hard. If it seems to demand too much effort to hold a picture in your mind, you might want to focus on self-talk alone. However, the more often you visualize, the easier it becomes, and learning to control your mind consciously in this way will not only help you to attract your goals, but will also improve your intuition.

You can visualize whatever you want to achieve, but to get the most out of visualization follow these rules:

• Visualize when you are relaxed: deep relaxation helps you to hold mental images for longer, and brings with it a positive outlook; this is because a completely relaxed body cannot hold destructive emotions. You can practice visualization at any time of day, but two of the best times are just after you wake up or just before going to sleep, when your mind and body are at their most relaxed.

• Repeat your visualization often: there are no rules about how often you should visualize. Some people put aside 15 minutes a day, others half an hour a week. Just remember that, to be effective, visualization should be repeated more than once.

• Make your visualization as real as possible: the more real you can make it, the more powerful it will be. Integrate into the visualization as many of the five senses as you can.

• Believe in your visualization: whatever the subject of your visualization, it is important to believe that it can come about in reality.

• Let your visualization go when you have finished: feel confident that your desire will be granted and let the thought go. Once your subconscious has a clear message about what you want, it will work with your conscious mind to inspire you in the right direction. Use the inspirations you receive in tandem with your plan of action.

### the power of self-talk

Like visualization, the words you use are continually sending messages to your subconscious about who you are and what you are capable of.

Talking to yourself positively is always a bonus, but you can also use self-talk in a more specific way—in the form of affirmations—to keep you on track with your detox and to bring your goals closer.

An affirmation is a statement, made in the present, about how you want your life to be. If you were to use an affirmation to attract a new car, you could say, "I now have a car that suits all my needs. It's attractive, reliable, and easily affordable." Putting your affirmation in the present tense stimulates your subconscious to connect you with what you want now instead of in the future.

To get an affirmation to work for you, you need to follow a few basic rules:

• Phrase your affirmation in the positive: instead of affirming something like, "I am not untidy," put it in the positive by affirming, "I am neat and organized." This gives a clearer message to your subconscious.

• Phrase your affirmation in the present: affirm that what you want is yours at this moment. For example, say to yourself, "I am now wealthy," even if you are not. If you put your affirmation in the future, you will never realize it because the future never comes.

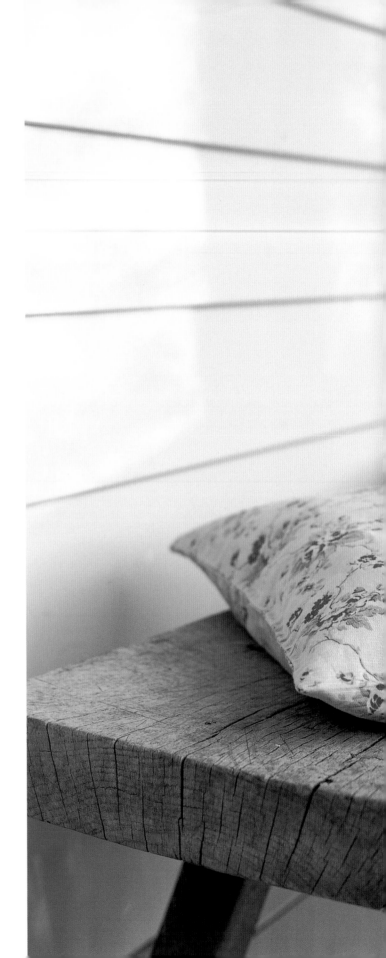

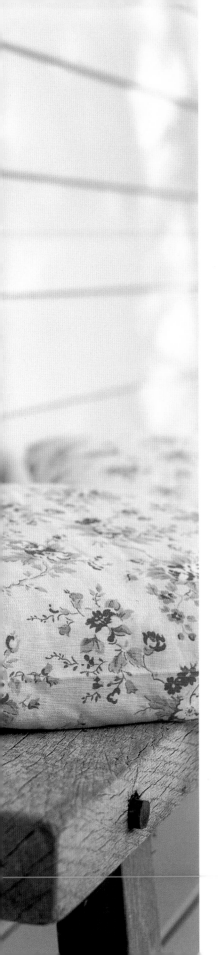

# visualization
## exercise

To experience for yourself how easy visualization can be, try the following exercise.

Find a quiet place where you won't be disturbed. Settle yourself into a comfortable position, either lying down or sitting, and close your eyes.

Relax by slowing down your breathing and gradually releasing any muscle tension.

Now imagine yourself in your own kitchen. Notice all the details. What time of day is it? Is your kitchen neat or in a mess? Run your hands along the counter. How does it feel? Pick up half a lemon that is lying on the counter, smell it. How strong is the smell? Then taste the lemon. Feel your mouth water as your tongue touches the bitterness.

When you have completed your visualization, say to yourself, "I feel wide awake and better than before," and open your eyes.

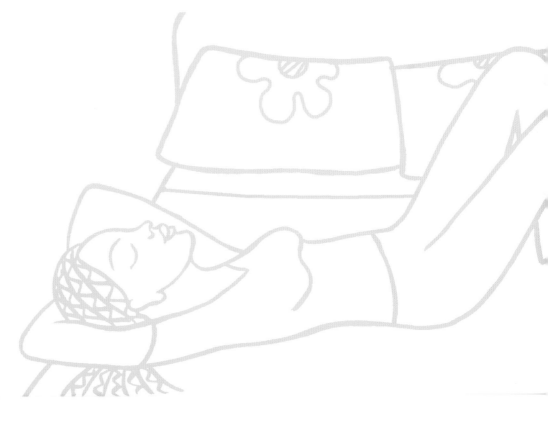

# meditation for
# dissolving barriers

If you sense that something is holding you back—preventing you from detoxing your mind and reaching your goals—try this meditation to dissolve the obstacle to your success.

Start by finding a quiet place where you are unlikely to be disturbed and make yourself comfortable. Take a few slow, deep breaths, and release any tension with the out breath.

Now imagine yourself being filled with feelings of confidence and success.

In front of you, imagine a path with an obstacle—any obstacle—blocking the way.

Say to yourself, "I have learned what I need to learn from this obstacle." Look at the obstacle and, as you do so, project a feeling of love. See the obstacle dissolving and disappearing.

Thank the obstacle for removing itself and then, feeling confident, move forward along the path, passing through the place where the obstacle was.

Now let the image fade. Feeling positive about what has occurred, say to yourself, "I feel confident. I am successful, and I have learned something from this obstacle. I can now move forward along my path happily and confidently."

Take a few deep breaths, feel your presence in your body, and open your eyes.

Acknowledge any insights that come to you after this meditation. For example, an insight could come in the form of an urge to connect with someone who could help you, or as a revelation about what you have learned from the obstacle.

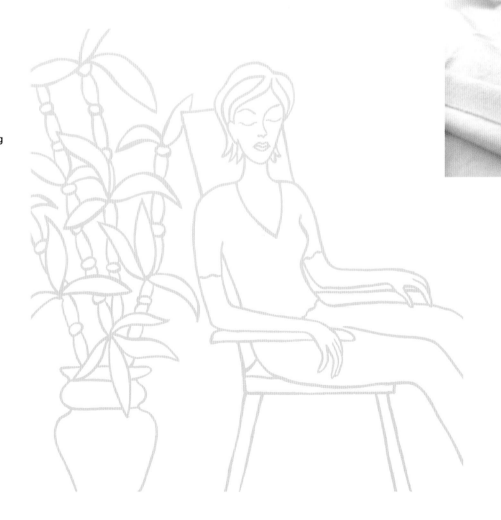

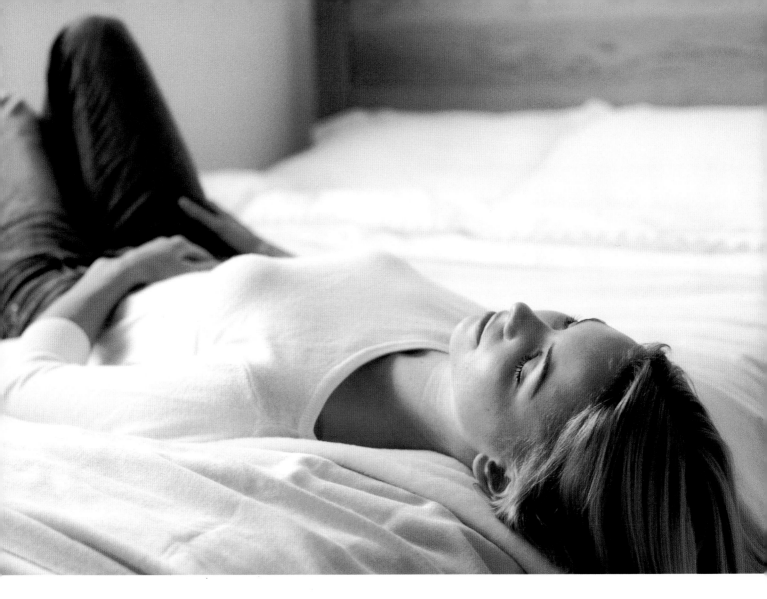

• Make your affirmation personal to you: the more specific your affirmation is to your life, the easier it will be to have confidence in it.

• Make your affirmation reasonable: there is no point affirming something that you don't believe will ever come about.

• Put some genuine feeling into your affirmation: speaking an affirmation with feeling and conviction gives it power.

• Repeat your affirmation often: say your affirmation to yourself either aloud or in your head on a regular basis. The more you say it to yourself, the more likely it is to work for you.

## when things don't come easily

There are occasions when you work with visualization and self-talk persistently, but see no results. Sometimes a particular outcome is just not right for you, or you may be subconsciously blocking the process. Here are some of the reasons why you may be sabotaging your efforts:

*You are holding onto old thoughts and emotional patterns.*

*You don't truly desire the object or situation.*

*You don't believe you deserve what you are asking for.*

*You don't believe you will get it.*

*You are worrying about it.*

# 4 take action

Now that you have paved the way
to success by doing the energy work,
put your plans into action and make
intuition part of your everyday life.

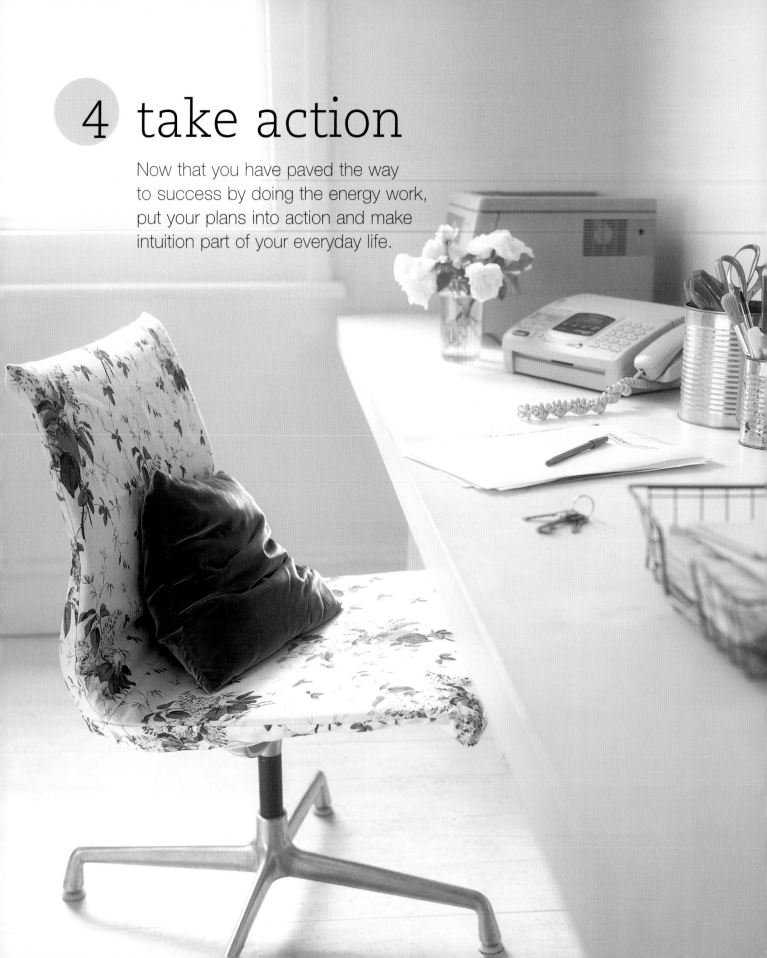

## positive habits

If you have completed step 2 (see pages 14–19), you will already have devised a goal plan and a detoxing program against which to measure your achievements, and you will probably also have worked out a timetable for each goal or task. The time frame that you have established is of course founded largely on guesswork, since tasks may take a longer or shorter time to complete than expected. However, there are a number of positive habits that you can adopt that will help you to maintain mental clarity and see both your goal plan and detox program through to a satisfactory conclusion:

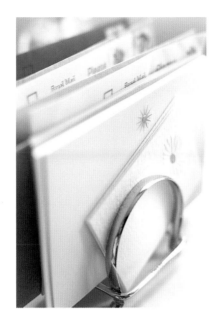

• Get organized: how often does it happen that you decide to make a telephone call, write a letter, or read an article, but find that, at the last moment, you just cannot lay your hands on the information needed to carry out the task?

Many people waste a vast amount of time looking for the things they need before they ever get around to taking action, so the advice here is to give top priority to the proper organization of your personal belongings. This means that everything should have a place and those things that you use frequently, such as pens, stamps, and diary, should be kept somewhere where they are easily accessible.

• Clear up: getting into the habit of putting things away immediately after you have used them will keep you organized and will save you a lot of "clearing-up time" and "looking-for-things time." Again, those things that are in frequent use should be easy to get at and easy to put away. If they are, it will encourage you to stay neat.

• Get moving: when you realize that it has become necessary to carry out a task, do it there and then. Individuals who procrastinate over the little things in life, such as dealing with letters, writing telephone numbers in an address book, or reading magazine articles, discover that it is all too easy to allow these seemingly trivial tasks to build up—and they end up needing to detox their lives!

• Cut out time-wasters: are there long-established patterns of behavior that you continue to repeat even though they no longer reap real benefits? Are there people whom you allow to take up your time when you would rather be doing something else? Do you spend time worrying unnecessarily or going over in your mind past events that you cannot do anything about? Look at how you spend your day and how you use your mind. Is there anyone or anything in your life that is robbing you of your time, energy, and clarity of thought?

• Stay focused: it is all too easy to dilute your energy and efforts by attempting to keep too many balls in the air at the same time—which leads you into a position where you are doing a little bit of everything but not finishing any task. Learn to pace yourself and set time limits to complete your tasks. Tell yourself that you will not move on to the next task until you have completed the one at hand.

## the best time to take action

If you need to be reassured about whether or not you should be pursing a particular course of action, the best policy is to follow your intuition. Most people have recognized an intuitive twinge at some point in their

# tuning in to 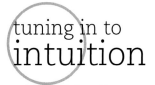intuition

Tuning in to your intuition is easy once you know how. Intuitive messages tend to be quiet and subtle, so you need a calm, clear mind to be aware of them.

This relaxation exercise will get you used to being in the right frame of mind to receive messages—until it becomes automatic. After a bit of practice you will be able to receive information no matter where you are or what you are doing.

Find a comfortable place to lie down. Shut your eyes, slow down your breathing, and think about relaxing your entire body. Starting with your toes, move up your body, relaxing each part as you go, until you feel calm and peaceful.

Imagine that your mind is totally empty. Ask your intuition about the situation you would like guidance on.

The idea is to be focused but relaxed, so don't try too hard. Allow any information to drift into your mind. Sometimes the answer will come immediately or you will get a clear physical indication. At other times you simply have to give the question to your intuition and expect to receive an answer within a couple of days. If you get no clear guidance, it is usually better to wait.

Answers can come in a number of ways, but if you feel that after a few days you have received no clear sign, do this exercise again and see if you have any further insights.

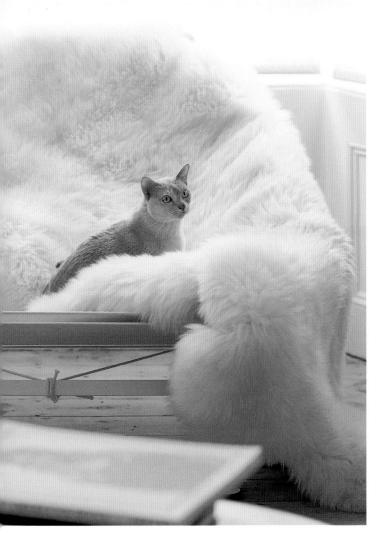

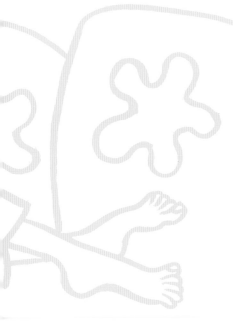

lives, whether it was a strong gut feeling that later paid off or simply an inner certainty that something was going to happen before it did.

Intuitive messages often take the form of feelings, ideas, and insights. We are especially susceptible to receiving information when our mind drifts off—when, for example, we are daydreaming, walking, having a bath, or falling asleep. It might be a physical feeling or a mental "click" when something feels just right.

It may be hard to tell whether a message comes from intuition or the intellect. Sometimes, when you ask your intuition for advice, your intellect jumps in with an obvious answer—an answer that may be based on fear, guilt, or a strong desire. Intuitive messages, on the other hand, are usually subtle and accompanied by a feeling of inner certainty. With practice it should become easier to tell the difference.

## putting intuition into practice

To benefit from your intuition you need to make it part of your everyday life. When you have to make a decision, run through the options in your mind and see how each of them makes you feel. If you take action only when your reactions are inviting and positive, you will need to apply less effort to achieve good results. If there is something you always feel negative about, ask your intuition what you could do to improve the situation. If you find yourself resisting doing something, ask yourself what you would rather do.

You can sometimes prevent negative situations from developing by paying attention to your feelings of irritability, resentment, or negativity and listening to the messages your intuition has to give you. If you find it difficult to "pick up" messages, try spending time in a tranquil environment, listening to soothing music, or carrying out some form of exercise. Doing these things should help you calm down emotionally, which will in turn make you more receptive.

# 5 let go of worries

An essential part of detoxing your mind is banishing
unhelpful thoughts—at least for a while. The aim
of this part of the detox program is to give your mind
a rest from everyday cares.

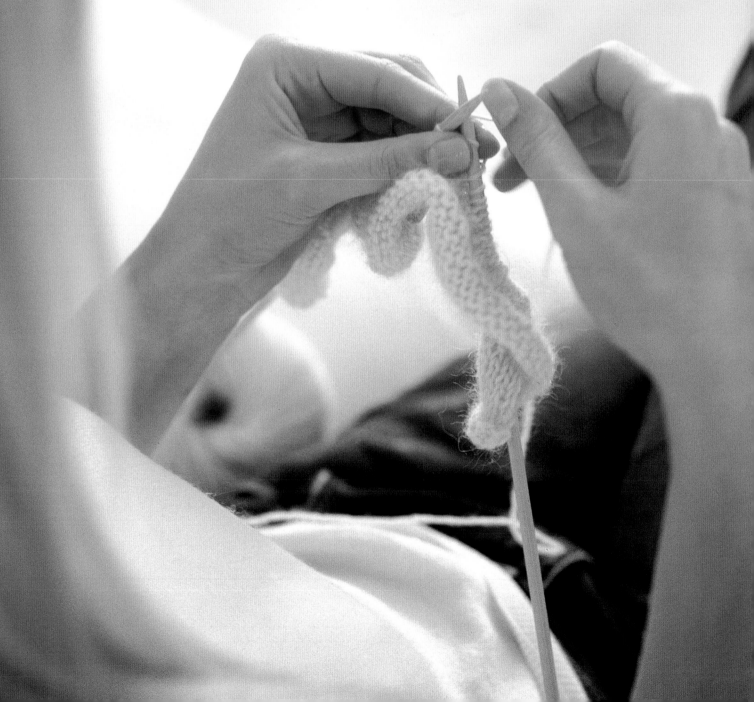

### saying goodbye to your worries

Meditating, having a relaxing bath, going for a walk—anything uplifting and relaxing will help you to let go of a problem. But sometimes you may feel that you don't deserve to relax or that, if you let your problem go even for a short time, you might not be able to resolve it. If you are in this frame of mind, try the meditation below.

When you have finished meditating, do something that will let your mental energy continue to flow in a relaxing way, such as watching an entertaining film or listening to music—anything that makes you feel good. Set a time limit for your break—maybe half an hour a day—and don't let yourself get bogged down in your problem until your time is up. Forgetting your problems for a while is good for your health as well as your mind. When your time is up, you can go back to your problem and address it with renewed clarity and inspiration.

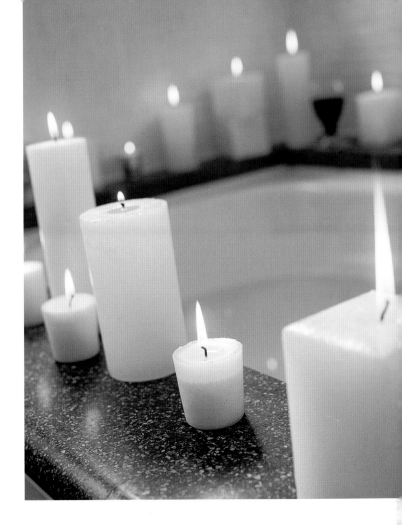

# meditation for
# letting go

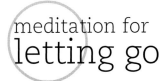

Before you do the meditation, write a description of whatever is troubling you. In this way, if you need to come back to your problem to resolve it at a later date, you have it on paper—so there is no reason why you cannot let it go for a short while.

Start by finding somewhere comfortable to sit or lie down where you won't be disturbed. Concentrate on slowing down your rate of breathing and consciously releasing tension from your body.

Now imagine a small rain cloud appearing in front of you in the sky and envisage yourself putting your problems into or on top of the cloud. You can fill it up with as many worries as you want to get rid of.

When you have finished and your mind feels empty, imagine the rain cloud floating off high into the sky.

As it floats away, say to yourself, "My problems are going off into the universe to be resolved. Answers will come back to me."

Watch the cloud floating away until it is a tiny dot and then see it disappear entirely.

See the sun coming out and enjoy the feel of its warmth. Be confident that you will receive the answers to your problems.

Now let the image fade.

Take a few slow deep breaths and open your eyes, saying to yourself, "I give myself permission to have a break from my problems."

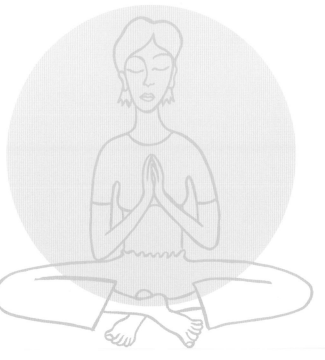

# do it now

Detoxing your mind is about changing your thinking
habits to suit your aims. It is about letting go of
behavior that sabotages your goals and learning to
replace it with skills that encourage clear thinking
and a strong belief in yourself.

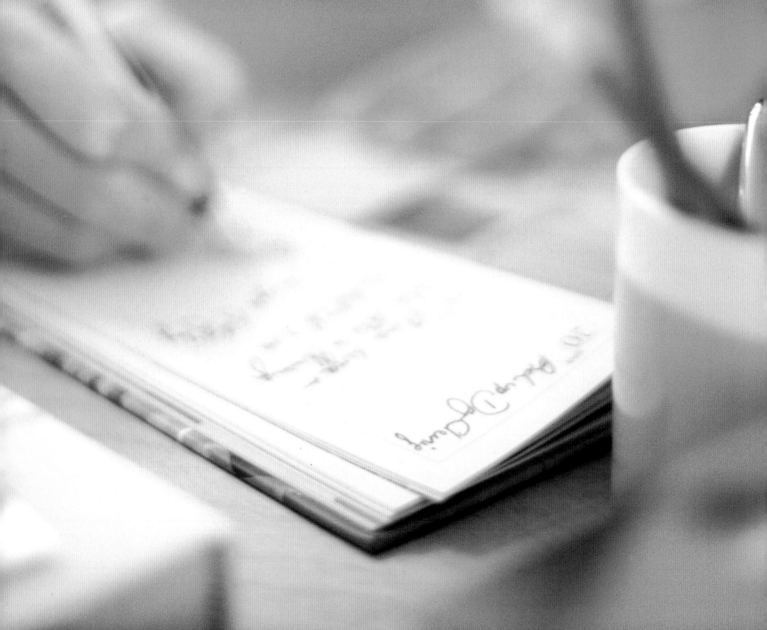

## mind tools

Knowing what you want to achieve, having a plan of action, using your imagination, being positive, organized and in tune with your intuition are all tools you need to detox your mind and achieve your goals.

## troubleshooting

*I have a tendency to put things off*
Motivate yourself by making a "to do" list. Then take one task and get on with it right now. If you don't have much time, make it something that can be completed quickly.

*My mind is overloaded*
Write down everything that's on your mind. If there is anything on the list that you can act on right now, do so.

*I am always worried about something*
Define what's bothering you, then decide whether you can do anything about it. If you can take action to resolve your worry, begin it now. If there's nothing you can do, give your mind a break by taking some exercise.

*I feel bad about myself*
Be clear about why you feel the way you do. If there is something you can do about it, do it now. Devise one or more affirmations that boost your self-esteem and say them to yourself frequently, particularly when you are feeling bad.

*I know I'm a scatterbrain*
Write down all the things you need to do and prioritize your list. Take action on something that you know you can finish in a short space of time. Promise yourself that you will work through your list, finishing each task before moving on to the next.

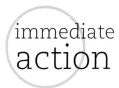

# immediate action

Over the next 24 hours, start taking note of your thoughts. What is your thinking style? Does your mind jump from one thought to another, or are you constantly preoccupied with something that needs to be done or something that's worrying you? Decide how you could change your thinking in a way that would make daily life run more smoothly or take the pressure off for a while.

if you cannot do anything to resolve a problem, it is pointless to dwell on it

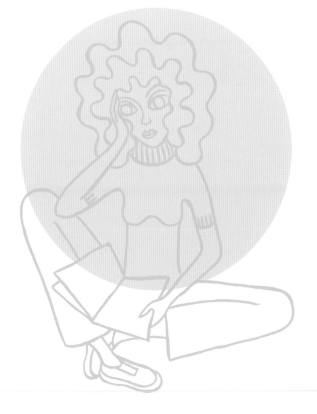

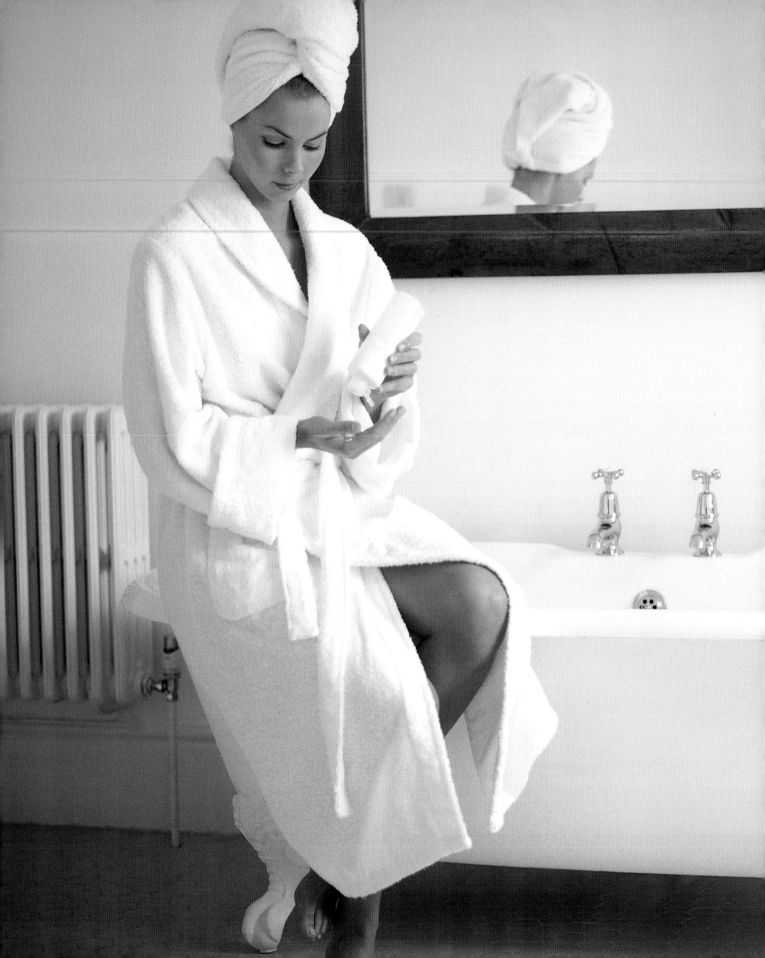

# detox
# your body

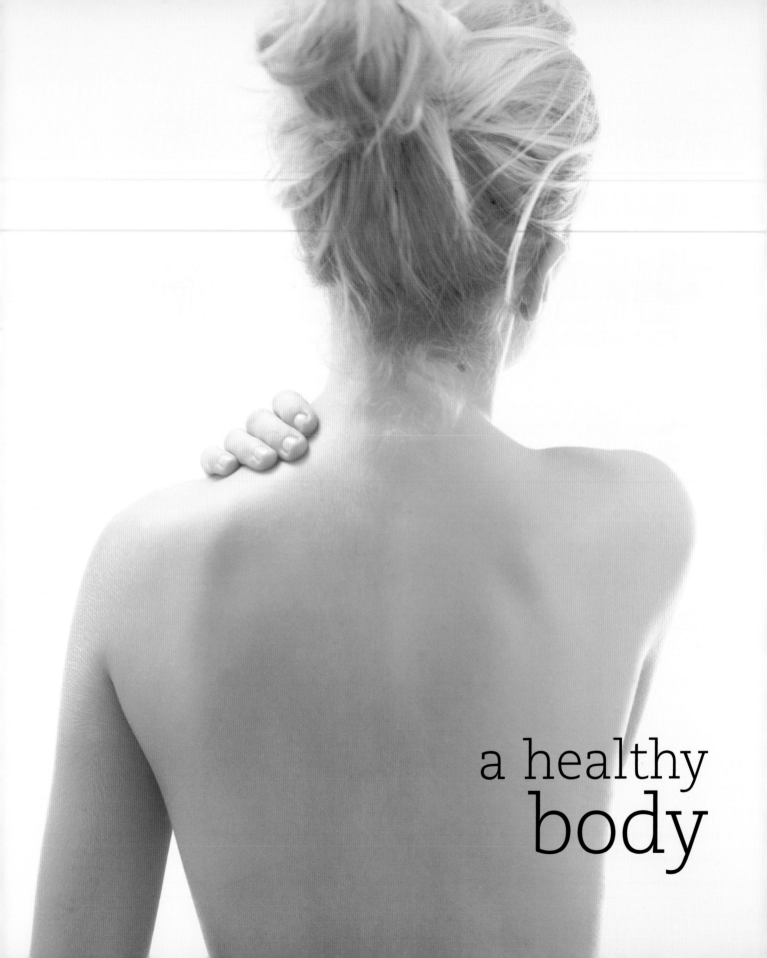

a healthy
body

Our bodies have to deal daily with a huge array of pollutants. We don't always get enough exercise or sleep. Processed foods, too much fat and sugar, caffeine and alcohol—all take their toll on health. If environmental and dietary toxins build up in the body, they contribute to fatigue, weight gain, allergies, headaches, skin eruptions, digestive disorders, slower mental processes, and a weakened immune system.

Fortunately, the body has its own purifying system, but if it becomes overworked and overloaded, a body detox may be the answer. Detoxing doesn't have to be hard or boring—you can have a short blast over a weekend or do it slowly and gradually over a couple of weeks.

There are many tools, such as herbs and essential oils, that make detoxing easier. There are treatments to rejuvenate tired skin and hair preparations that bring out your hair's natural shine. By using these tools, combined with a detox diet, regular exercise, and better-quality sleep, you will not only expel the toxins from your body, but also increase your energy, lift your mood, and feel more attractive.

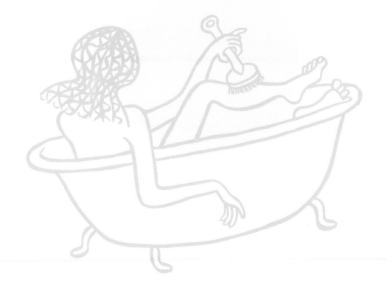

# 1 eat well

A balanced diet is the only way to make sure your body gets what it requires for optimum health. This means consuming food and drink that fulfills nutritional needs and allows your body to maintain its normal functions.

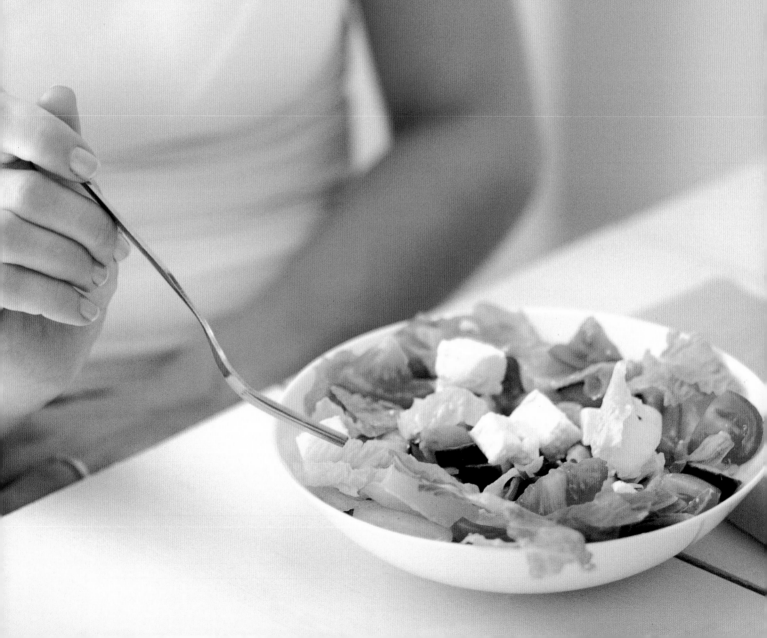

# strategy
## for healthy eating

- eat regularly

- eat plenty of fresh fruit and vegetables

- choose fresh, whole foods—the nearer foods are to their natural state, the more nutritious they are

- keep fats and oils to a minimum, aiming mainly for unsaturated fats

- choose low-fat varieties of dairy products, lean meat, and any type of fish

- vary your diet

- limit your intake of caffeine and alcohol

- keep treats such as chocolate, cakes, cookies, and chips to a minimum

- drink plenty of water (see pages 40–41)

start a detox diet at a time when you feel confident and relatively free from stress

## a balanced diet

There is increasing evidence that what we eat profoundly affects physical and mental wellbeing, and that following a balanced diet is crucial to optimal health. Experts say that such a diet consists of 55 percent carbohydrates, 30 percent fats, and 15 percent proteins. It should also be rich in fibre, vitamins and minerals.

- Carbohydrates are converted into glucose for the body to use as energy. Cut down on simple carbohydrates such as white and brown sugar, which provide a quick burst of energy. Increase complex carbohydrates, which are digested more slowly and release glucose more gradually, resulting in steadier energy levels; brown rice, wholewheat or rye bread, brown pasta, granola, and oatmeal are all highly beneficial foods in this group.

- Fats provide the body with the most concentrated source of energy. They also help the body to absorb the fat-soluble vitamins A, D, and E, and provide essential fatty acids (unsaturated fats), which are vital for the healthy functioning of the heart, nerves, hormones, and immune system. Good sources include oily fish, cold-pressed seed or vegetable oils, nuts, and seeds.

- Proteins are needed for cell growth and are used to make enzymes, hormones, and antibodies. They are made up of amino acids, some of which cannot be created by the body and must be obtained from the diet. Lean meat, fish, and eggs provide high-quality proteins. These should be balanced with vegetable proteins from soy beans, lentils, tofu, and nuts.

- Fiber provides the bulk for food to move through the body, aiding the process of digestion and elimination. Foods rich in fiber include whole-wheat bread, brown rice, wholegrain cereals, whole-wheat pasta, oatbran, vegetables, fresh and dried fruit, legumes, and nuts.

- Vitamins and minerals, found in all food groups, keep the body systems healthy and fight off disease. Water-soluble vitamins (the B vitamins and vitamin C) are not stored in the body and need to be obtained daily from food. Fat-soluble vitamins (A, D, E, and K) can be stored in the body for when they are needed.

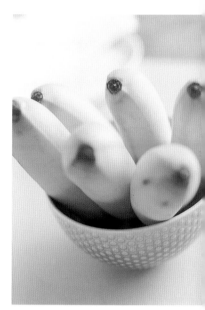

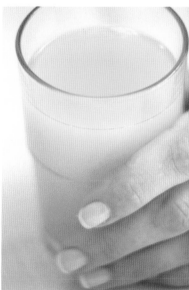

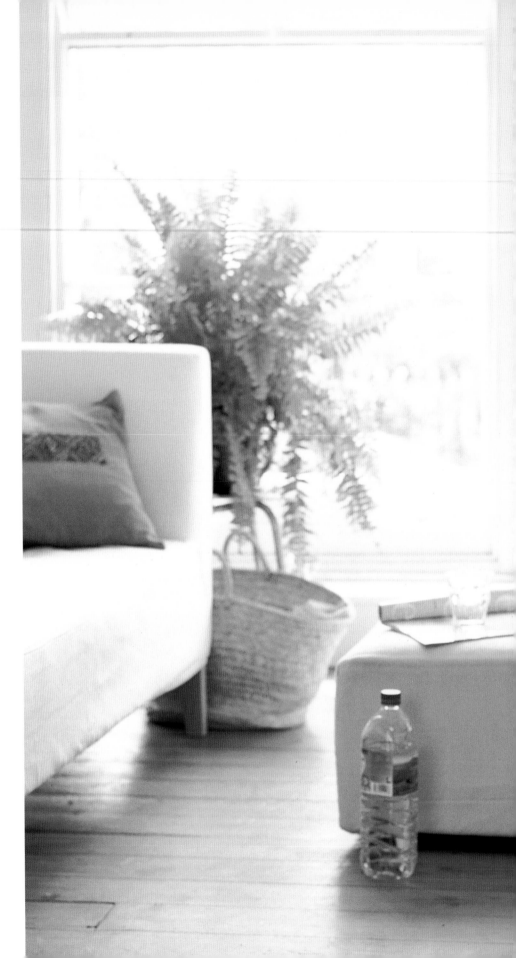

# drink more
# water

For optimal health, drink eight glasses of filtered water a day, equivalent to about 5 pints (2 litres). When detoxing, aim to increase water intake by following these tips:

• have a glass of water first thing in the morning when you wake up and in the evening before going to bed

• keep a bottle of water within easy reach during the day

• increase your intake of fresh fruit and vegetables; both have a high water content as well as many other health benefits

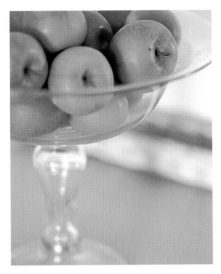
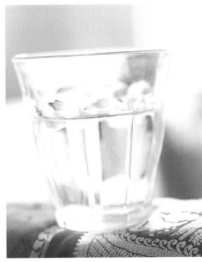
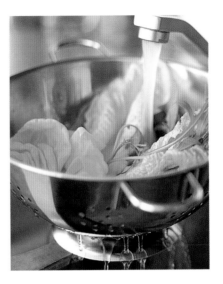

## what a detox diet involves

Deciding to embark on a detox diet is a positive way to kick-start your journey to a healthier lifestyle. Limiting the type of food and drink you consume for a temporary period gives your body a respite from unwholesome foods and chemicals, allowing its natural systems, in particular the liver and kidneys, to cleanse your body of unwanted substances. This is especially valuable if you suffer from an ailment such as irritable bowel syndrome, hay fever, or general sluggishness.

The focus of a detox diet is to cut down on or cut out those foods and drinks that build up toxins in your body and concentrate instead on those foods that help to cleanse your system. It can be anything from a short-term fasting detox, in which only water and one type of fruit is consumed, to a gentle cutting down of foods and drinks that cause stress to your system, which can be carried out over a period of several weeks.

The type of regime suitable for you depends on your reasons for wanting to detox, the time you have available, your general health, and your personality.

Where possible, choose organically grown food, which contains no residues from artificial pesticides and fertilizers, and has been produced without preservatives.

Do not embark on a detox diet if you are pregnant, breastfeeding, or unwell. People with long-standing medical conditions, those taking prescription medication, and those with diabetes or low blood sugar should also avoid detox diets, as should anyone who is suffering from a toxic build-up caused by long-term misuse of drugs or alcohol. If in doubt, seek the advice of your doctor.

## the power of $H_2O$

Water forms about 60 percent of body weight and is needed for every chemical reaction in the body; without enough water our bodies cannot function efficiently. If we are even slightly dehydrated, it can affect how good we feel mentally, emotionally, and physically, and how well we are able to work. Water plays a vital role in helping us to feel more satisfied by food. It helps to absorb and transport nutrients, vitamins, and minerals, and to flush out the waste from our system. When detoxing, the level of toxins released by our bodies is higher than normal, so we need to drink even more water than usual.

Although production of tap water is strictly regulated, it is advisable to use filtered water for both drinking and cooking throughout any detox diet. This should help to cut down on any toxins that may be found in tap water.

If you prefer to drink bottled water, compare the labels of different brands and choose a still water with a relatively low mineral and sodium content. Some sources of spring water are treated to meet hygiene standards, so they may not necessarily be better than filtered water.

# weekend detox diet

A weekend detox is ideal if you don't have the time or willpower to follow a strict regime for long. Remember to use filtered water for drinking and cooking during the detox. Any herbal tea is allowed through the weekend. It is wise to precede a two-day detox with a few days of gradual adjustment. For example, if you smoke or drink alcohol, start to cut back on coffee and convenience foods. In this way, when you start the full detox, you are less likely to get unpleasant side effects. Similarly, when the weekend is over, do not immediately go back to your old habits. With any luck, your liver will be cleaner, but it may also be more sensitive to the usual toxins.

## day one

### on waking

1 glass of hot water with a
 squeeze of fresh lemon juice

### breakfast

a large bowl of fresh fruit: apple,
 kiwi, berries, and grapes

### midmorning

1 glass of water

1 small carton of natural soy
 or goat milk yogurt with
 ½ teaspoon honey

### lunch

carrot and ginger soup:
2 large carrots, peeled and sliced
1 teaspoon chopped fresh ginger
1 large mug of water
sea salt
freshly ground black pepper
*Put the carrots and ginger in a saucepan. Cover with water and bring to a boil. Simmer until the carrots are tender. Let cool, then purée in a blender. Season with salt and pepper and serve.*

### midafternoon

1 glass of water

2 oat crackers with
 thinly spread hummus

### supper

avocado salad:
1 avocado, sliced
2 large handfuls of mixed spinach,
 watercress, and arugula
½ small onion
2 tomatoes
1 tablespoon sunflower seeds
1 tablespoon pumpkin seeds
dressing:
1 tablespoon extra virgin olive oil
1 teaspoon cider vinegar
1 small garlic clove, finely chopped
sea salt
freshly ground black pepper
*Put the ingredients for the dressing in a large salad bowl and add the arugula, spinach, watercress, rocket, onion, and tomatoes. Toss the salad in the dressing and sprinkle with the seeds.*

baked apple dessert:
1 medium cooking apple,
 washed and cored
1 tablespoon chopped dates
1 tablespoon chopped almonds
2 tablespoons water
*Put the apple in a small baking dish and stuff the center with the dates and almonds. Add water. Bake in a preheated oven at 350°F (175°C) until the flesh is soft.*

### before bed

1 cup of camomile tea

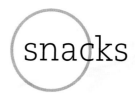

## snacks

**If you feel hungry between meals, try one of the following snacks. One teaspoon of spirulina (mineral-rich algae) in water before lunch will help to stop cravings.**

• a handful of dried apricots

• a couple of rice cakes with hummus

• a bowl of plain popcorn popped in olive oil

## day two

### on waking

1 glass of hot water with a
squeeze of fresh lemon juice

### breakfast

apple fruit smoothie:
1 glass of fresh apple juice
1 banana
1 small bowl of fresh fruit:
strawberries, raspberries,
blueberries, peaches, or apricots
*Purée in a blender, then serve.*

### midmorning

1 glass of water

2 oat crackers with
thinly spread hummus

### lunch

1 glass of water

warm spiced grapefruit:
1 pink grapefruit, halved,
with visible seeds removed
pinch of ground ginger
pinch of ground cinnamon
pinch of ground cloves
*Loosen grapefruit segments by
cutting between and around them
with a small knife. Sprinkle with
ginger, cinnamon, and cloves and
put under a preheated broiler for
5–10 minutes or until warm.*

grilled fresh fish (any kind) or
goat cheese
a large green salad, sprinkled with
sunflower seeds and pine nuts
a bag of sprouted alfalfa/mung beans
(available from natural-food stores)

### midafternoon

1 glass of water

1 small carton of natural soy
or goat milk yogurt with
½ teaspoon honey

### supper

basil and tomato soup:
3 large tomatoes, washed and
peeled
1 garlic clove, crushed
1 tablespoon fresh basil, chopped
a squeeze of lemon juice
*Put the tomatoes in a saucepan and
completely cover with boiling water.
Leave them for exactly 1 minute,
then slit the skins with a knife. The
skin should peel off easily. Put the
tomatoes and garlic in a blender and
purée until smooth. Transfer to a
saucepan and add the basil and
lemon. Simmer gently, then serve.*

an ear of corn with extra virgin olive
oil and freshly ground black pepper

### before bed

1 cup of camomile tea

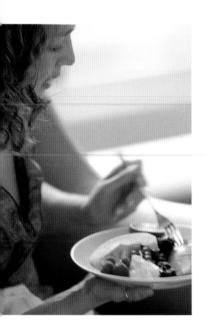

# two-week detox

A two-week general detox focuses on making simple alterations to your everyday eating habits rather than embarking on sweeping changes.

### reducing a build-up of toxins

If a short detox does not appeal to you, or if your usual diet is rich in alcohol, caffeine, and processed food, you may decide that you want to detox your body in a more gentle and flexible way over a two-week period or longer.

A longer-term detox involves cutting down or cutting out particular foods and drinks from your diet, including dairy products and processed foods (see opposite) and increasing your intake of water, vegetables, and fruit, and other detox superfoods (see page 47). The aim is to boost your overall health and encourage your body to eliminate old toxins that have accumulated over time.

It should go without saying that smoking is banned during any detox regime. There are around 2,000 chemicals found in cigarette smoke, some of which are the hardest for the body to process.

### dairy products

Ideally, all dairy products, including butter, cheese, and yogurt, should be eliminated from your diet during a two-week detox because many people find that cows' milk products cause bloating, discomfort, and excess mucus in the sinuses.

Organic goat or sheep milk products are acceptable in moderation as part of a detox diet because their process of fermentation makes them easier to digest than cows' milk. Almond and rice milks are suitable alternatives, and soy milk and other soybean products can also be used, but choose organic, unsweetened brands.

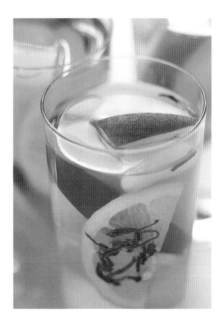

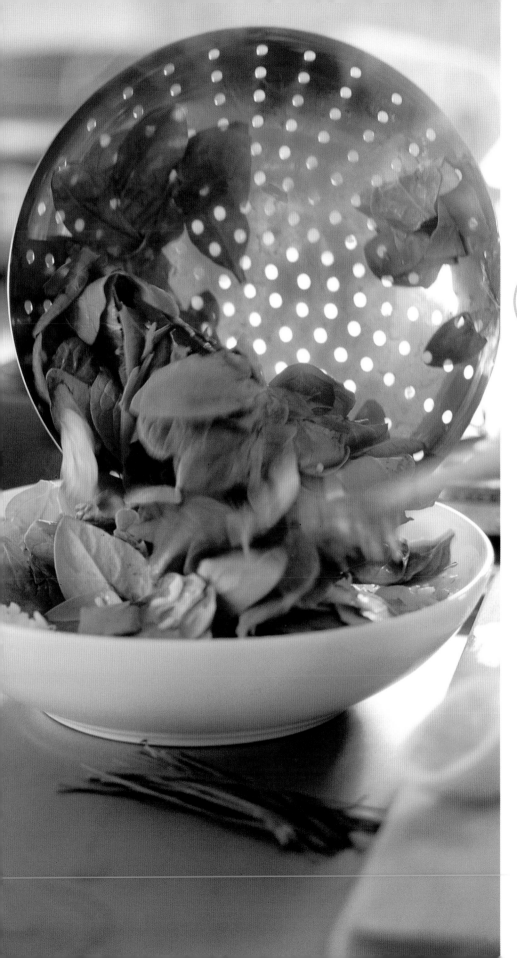

# foods to avoid

For a two-week period, cut down or cut out your intake of any or all of the following:

• dairy products and margarines

• refined carbohydrates (white rice, white pasta, white bread)

• prepackaged, processed food (canned foods, packet foods, and ready-meals)

• sugar (brown and white), candy, and chocolate

• tea and coffee

• alcohol

• carbonated drinks and squashes

• pastries and cookies

• deep-fried foods

• red meat

### fruit and vegetables

Fresh fruit and vegetables are an excellent source of nutrients, and many are rich in antioxidants, substances that protect the body from harm by unstable molecules called free radicals. Although free radicals are produced as part of normal cell processes, they can be increased by environmental toxins and stress. In extreme cases, free radicals can cause ailments such as heart disease and cancer. Aim to eat four portions of fruit and four of vegetables daily, and vary your choice to get a good mix of vitamins, minerals, and antioxidants.

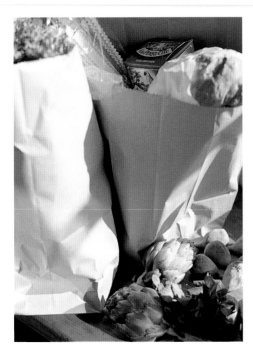

### whole grains

Whole grains provide fiber, vitamins (especially B and E), minerals, and complex carbohydrates. Brown rice is very effective in helping to expel waste from the body. Quinoa, a small protein-rich grain with a nutty flavor, contains fiber, magnesium, iron, and several B vitamins, and can be used instead of pasta or mixed into salads. Oats provide B vitamins and magnesium, and help promote a healthy nervous system. Millet, barley, rice cakes, oat crackers, and rye bread are also beneficial forms of grain to include in your detox. Give your body a rest from wheat, especially if you are prone to bloating.

### side effects

Among the side effects of a detox diet are headaches, loose bowels, constipation, fuzzy-headedness, a furry tongue, and skin outbreaks. Headaches are common if you are used to drinking caffeine. If you get a headache, drink lots of water and lie down for a while before using painkillers. Increasing your intake of brown rice can boost the elimination of toxins and reduce side effects. Reducing citrus fruit such as oranges and grapefruit can also help, since these fruits are very aggressive cleansers. Finally, try to get as much rest as possible.

## additions
### to a detox diet

Multivitamin supplements help to maintain levels of essential nutrients. Other supplements that can be beneficial in a long-term detox include kelp, milk thistle, cranberry, and linseed.

• kelp helps to balance metabolic rate; it is particularly useful when you are changing your diet

• milk thistle boosts liver function

• cranberry boosts kidney function

• linseed helps eliminate toxins; soak 1 tablespoon in water overnight and take before breakfast

• a probiotic such as acidophilus will help create a healthy gut environment

# detox superfoods

During a two-week detox, you should aim to increase your intake of water, fruits, vegetables, and herbs, whole grains, legumes and beans, nuts and seeds, and some oils. Many fruits and vegetables are particularly good at helping the body with the detoxing processes; they are high in water and packed full of essential vitamins and minerals. Aim to eat fruit and vegetables as fresh as possible, and try to consume a high percentage of them raw, since raw food is not only higher in nutrients, but it also helps to clean the gut more efficiently than cooked food. Wherever possible, choose organic produce, which should be less taxing for your body to process.

| food or drink | comments | beneficial effects |
|---|---|---|
| water | 4–5 pints (1½–2 litres) is the recommended daily intake of water; increase this during a detox diet, especially after exercise or if the weather is hot | flushes out water-soluble toxins from your body |
| vegetables | useful detox vegetables include artichoke, asparagus, beets, broccoli, cabbage (red and white), carrot, celery, garlic, onion, tomato, watercress | support the liver and kidneys, help to cleanse the blood and improve bowel function; aim to have four portions of vegetables daily when detoxing |
| fruits | useful detox fruits include apple, apricot (fresh and dried), cranberry, grapes (red and white), lemon, orange, papaya | support the liver and kidneys, help to cleanse the blood and improve bowel function; aim to have four portions daily |
| herbs and spices | useful detox herbs include basil, chives, coriander, garlic, marjoram, oregano, parsley, rosemary, sage, thyme; spices such as ginger, dill, caraway, and fennel seeds aid digestion | many fresh herbs have specific detoxing effects; they can be used in cooking, added to salads, or steeped in hot water to make herbal teas (see pages 62–63) |
| whole grains | useful detox whole grains include brown rice, oats, millet, barley, quinoa, rice cakes, oat crackers, rye bread | provide fiber, vitamins, minerals, complex carbohydrates, which maintain blood sugar levels, preventing cravings and drops in energy levels |
| pulses and beans | useful detox legumes and beans include lentils; garbanza, kidney, lima, haricot, borlotti and flageolet beans | great fillers that are a good source of protein, complex carbohydrates, fiber, vitamins, and minerals |
| seeds and nuts | useful detox seeds and nuts include linseed, pumpkin seeds, sunflower seeds, sesame seeds, walnuts, brazil nuts | good source of protein, minerals, and essential fatty acids; aim to eat 1 tablespoon of nuts or seeds, or a mixture, daily |
| oils | useful oils include cold-pressed oils made from seeds or nuts such as flaxseed (linseed), walnut, sesame, and sunflower; virgin olive oil | aim to have 2 tablespoons of unheated oil daily; unsaturated fats have a delicate chemical structure and once oil is heated, for example in frying, unhealthy substances form |
| seaweeds | useful seaweeds, also known as sea vegetables, include nori, arame, kelp, kombu, and wakame | a good vegetable source of protein that helps to eliminate heavy metals from the body; toast nori sheets until crisp and sprinkle onto salads; soak arame and mix into salads |

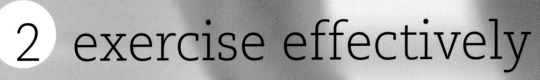

# 2 exercise effectively

Exercise is an essential part of a detox program. Not only does it build strength, boost energy levels and help reduce stress, but it is also a good way to help release toxins, burn calories, and keep you in good shape.

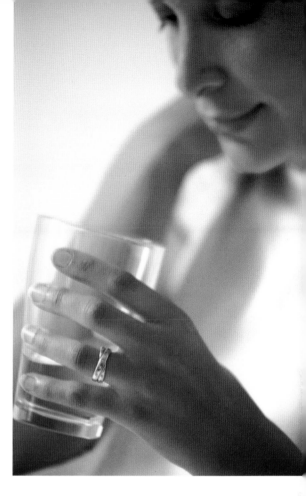

# warm up
## and cool down

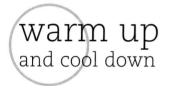

**Start each exercise session with a warm-up period of 5–10 minutes. This will help you stretch your muscles slowly and allow you to increase your level of activity gradually. For example, begin walking slowly and then steadily increase the pace. After you have finished exercising, leave 5–10 minutes for cooling down. Again, this will let you stretch your muscles and allow your heart rate to slow down gradually, helping to prevent injury.**

### types of exercise

For the purposes of a body detox, exercise has been divided into two categories: aerobic exercise and spot exercises. The aim of aerobic exercise is to get your heart pumping and to eliminate toxins from your system, while spot exercises (see pages 50–51) are designed to tone particular parts of your body. If you are aware of any health reason why you might not be able to exercise safely, consult your doctor before beginning a new exercise program.

### aerobic exercise

Ideally, you should do some type of aerobic exercise— fast walking, jogging, swimming, dancing, or bicycling —for 20 minutes at least three times a week. While exercise is a crucial part of any detox program because it helps release toxins from your body, you should aim to incorporate this amount of aerobic exercise into your life whether or not you are detoxing.

Choose an activity that you enjoy and that you can build up slowly and gradually. Walking is popular because it is easy to incorporate into most people's schedules and does not require special equipment.

Start with manageable, attainable exercise goals. Setting your goals too high can be frustrating, and can lead quickly to injuries or "burn out." If you are not used to exercising, start slowly, and give yourself time to increase your stamina. If you persevere, you will quickly notice results.

Make sure you increase your water intake when you exercise, since your body will be releasing more fluids.

## a simple routine

The five exercises described below are designed to address the essential problem areas: the waist, the abdomen, the buttocks, the thighs, and the upper arms and chest. If you get into the habit of doing the exercises every day, they will help to keep your body toned and flexible. Repeat each exercise up to eight times to begin with, increasing the number as you build stamina.

## preparation for exercise

Before starting each exercise session, march on the spot for a couple of minutes. Roll your shoulders forward and backward five times, and turn your head from one side to the other five times. Then, keeping your knees soft, gently bend forward, sideways, and backward from the waist five times. Grasp your hands behind your back and lift for a few seconds to stretch your shoulders.

To stretch your thighs, stand up and, bending one leg behind you, grasp the ankle and bring it up toward your buttocks for a few seconds, then change to the other leg. Finish by shaking out your arms and legs.

This sequence will help to warm up your body. After you have finished, repeat the sequence to cool down.

### waist slimmer

1  Stand with your feet parallel to each other, hip width apart, and knees slightly bent.
2  Put your hands on your shoulders. The shoulders should be relaxed and the elbows straight out to the sides.
3  With your back and neck straight, and abdominal muscles pulled in, turn your upper body from the waist around to the right, keeping your hips straight, then turn it back to the center.
4  Turn your upper body around to the left, keeping hips straight, then turn it back to the center.

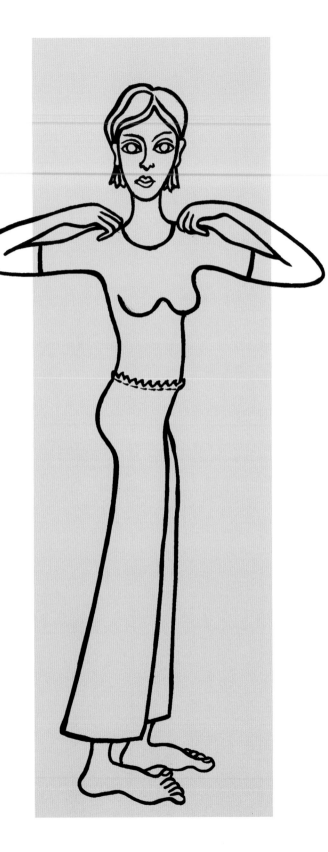

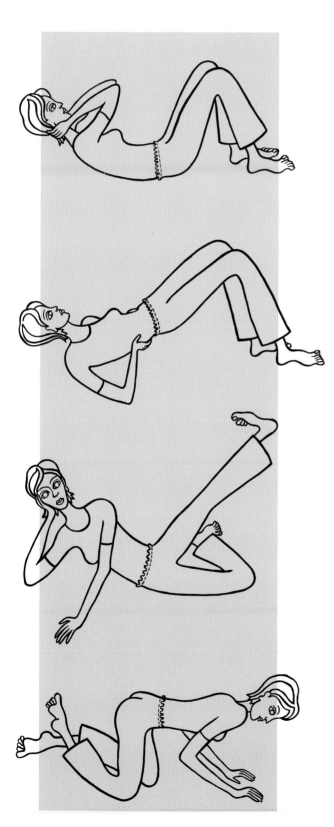

### stomach flattener

1 Lie on your back with knees bent and feet parallel to each other, hip width apart.

2 Put your hands behind your head, elbows pointing out.

3 Breathe in and press your lower back into the ground.

4 Breathe out and lift your shoulders and upper back up toward the ceiling, taking care not to strain your neck or your back. As your head rises, keep your lower back against the floor and pull in your abdominal muscles.

5 Breathe in as you gently lower your upper back and shoulders to the floor and release your abdominal muscles.

### bottom tightener

1 Lie on your back with knees bent and feet parallel to each other, hip width apart.

2 Pull in your stomach and, keeping the upper part of your body on the ground, push your pelvis and buttocks upward, either using your hands for support or keeping them by your sides. Then squeeze your buttocks and pull up your pelvic floor tightly.

3 Hold the position and alternately tighten and release the muscles eight times before lowering your buttocks to the floor.

### thigh toner

1 Lie on the floor on your right side with both legs straight. Prop yourself up on your right elbow with your head resting on your hand. Bend your right leg, so that your right foot is behind you, keeping both thighs straight. Rest your left hand flat on the floor in front of you with arm straight to act as a support.

2 Lift your left leg into the air, keeping it straight and facing forward. Push out your heel so that your toes are pointing toward your nose. (*Please follow written the instructions carefully; this movement has been only loosely represented by the artist*.)

3 Lower your leg, then lift it again. After doing this exercise ten times, turn onto your left side and repeat with the right leg.

### arm and chest strengthener

1 Kneel on all fours with your hands parallel to each other on the floor in front of you, palms down and shoulder width apart. Keep your arms straight and at right angles to the floor.

2 Lift your feet in the air, crossing your ankles. Your back should be straight and your body supported by your arms and knees.

3 Breathe in as you bend your elbows and lower your chest to the floor. As in a press-up, your chest should not actually come into contact with the floor.

4 Breathe out as you push back up to your starting position.

# 3 enjoy your sleep

Adequate sleep is vital to wellbeing. It gives your body an opportunity for rest and renewal, and is particularly important at times when your physical systems are working hard to clear out toxins.

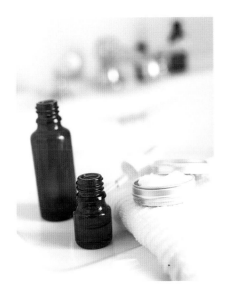

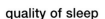

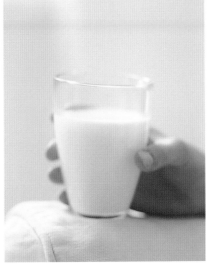

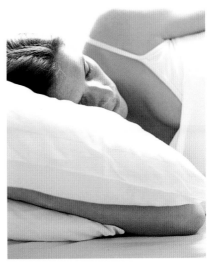

## quality of sleep

A good night's sleep can lift your mood, improve your mental and physical performance, and refresh your looks. The amount of sleep you need is dictated by your personal body clock, but if you are not sure how much sleep you need, aim for about eight hours. It is not unusual to become sleep-deprived from time to time as a result of everyday pressures, but if you find yourself continuously fatigued through lack of sleep, you may want to find out why. There are four main areas that can affect quality of sleep.

• Where you sleep: a bedroom that is too noisy, too light, too hot, or too cold can make it impossible to get a good night's sleep. Consider whether your mattress is as comfortable as it should be.

• Diet and exercise routine: a balanced diet and regular exercise encourage sleep. Exercising late at night or drinking too much caffeine or alcohol can disrupt sleep.

• Stress levels: worry—either about problems in your daily life or about whether you are getting enough sleep—can make sleep more elusive.

• Medical problems: if you are physically uncomfortable or feel unwell, the quality of your sleep will suffer.

## a sleep diary

Keep a sleep diary to monitor the time you spend sleeping and the quality of your sleep, along with factors that might be disturbing your sleep patterns. If you don't know why you can't sleep properly and there seems to be no improvement over time, seek advice from your doctor.

## tips for better sleep

• Relax in a warm bath: take time to relax your muscles and calm your mind by enjoying a warm, soothing bath.

• Release your worries: you can do this by writing down your worries and concerns before going to sleep. Give yourself permission to let go and sleep with a clear mind.

• Listen to relaxing music: classical music or any music that you find soothing and relaxing will do. Don't listen to music that arouses your emotions.

• Unwind with a guided journey: any mediation or hypnosis tape that relaxes you or enhances sleep should help you to wind down and clear your mind.

• Have a soothing drink: sipping a milky drink or a sleep-enhancing herbal drink will help to calm your body and mind and put you in the mood for sleep.

# 4 purify from the outside

You can encourage your body to release toxins by paying special attention to skin and hair. Exfoliating, bathing in sea salt, and self-massage all contribute to the process of physical purification.

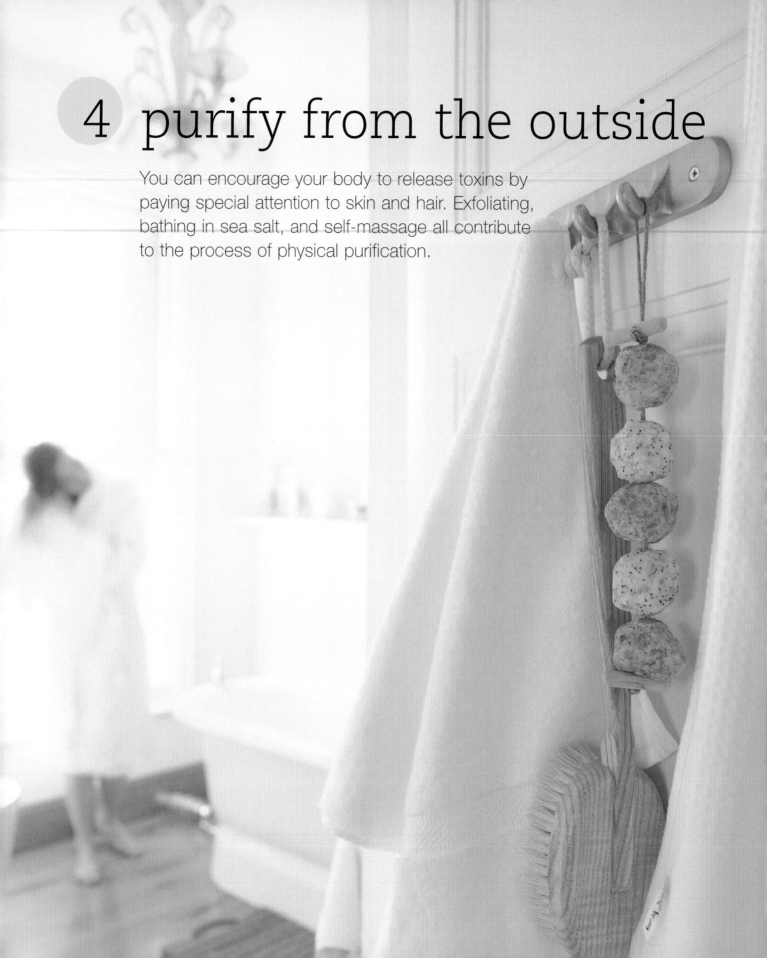

## soak yourself in
# sea salt

Taking a bath with sea salt will encourage elimination of toxins through the skin. Add the following salt and oils to a warm bath and soak in it for at least 20 minutes:

- 1 handful of sea salt
- 3 drops of lemon essential oil
- 3 drops of grapefruit essential oil
- 3 drops of lavender essential oil

### refresh your skin

Exfoliating helps to remove dead cells from your skin, cleans your pores, and allows your skin to breathe properly. The stimulating action of exfoliating improves blood and lymph circulation as well as the appearance of skin. Any kind of exfoliant will do. You could choose a loofah, a glove, or a brush, ideally one made from natural fibers. Exfoliating is very satisfying to do in the morning in the shower, before adding salt to the bath, or before a massage.

Beginning with your feet, gently work the loofah, glove, or brush up your legs in long sweeping strokes. Then, starting with your hands, move up your arms before attending to the lower part of your torso, moving upward toward your heart.

The process of exfoliation should take no more than 5 minutes, and you should do it once or twice a week. If you feel that it is making your skin sore, or your skin stings when you apply oil or cream afterward, you may be exfoliating too vigorously or too often, so stop doing it for a while.

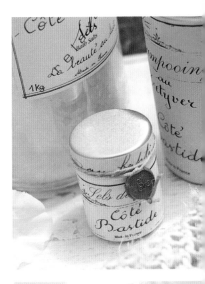

### cleanse your face

Use a simple face mask to unblock your pores and improve your complexion. Gently heat 4 tablespoons of oatmeal with half a cup of water until it resembles a paste. Leave to cool and mix in 2 tablespoons of honey. Smooth the mask thickly onto your face, avoiding the eye area, and leave for 20 minutes. Then rinse off with plenty of warm water and pat your face dry.

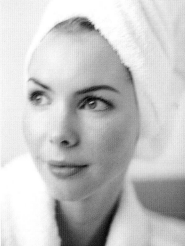

### rejuvenate your hair

To detox your hair and leave it shiny and feeling fresh, follow this routine. First shampoo and rinse your hair thoroughly. Put four camomile teabags in a bowl with 1 tablespoon of fresh rosemary. Pour over 1 pint (half a litre) of boiling water. Leave to cool for 15 minutes, then add 1 tablespoon of cider vinegar. Remove the teabags and the rosemary by pouring the liquid through a strainer, then pour the strained liquid over your hair. Massage it into your scalp and rinse out thoroughly with plenty of clean warm water.

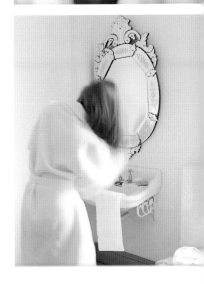

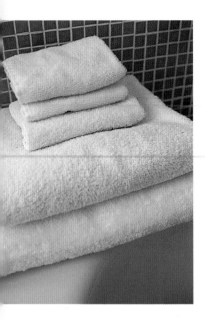

### self-massage

Massage enhances the effectiveness of a detox by improving circulation and helping your body to release toxins. Self-massage can be particularly useful if you suffer from fatigue, insomnia, muscle tension, circulatory disorders, or skin problems. You can massage yourself slowly and gently, to encourage relaxation and improve circulation, or you can massage yourself quickly, with more pressure, to counteract fatigue. Be very careful when massaging any areas that look red or are sore.

### body massage

Sit on a bed or in a comfortable chair. You can either massage your whole body—allow about 20 minutes—or pick an area of your body you would like to focus on.

If you are doing your whole body, start with your feet and move upward. Then give attention to your hands, moving upward, followed by your torso and, last, your face. The idea is to work toward the heart. On the right are the techniques you can use. You should work in the way that feels right to you.

### giving yourself a facial massage

Wash your hands. Add 2 drops of rose essential oil and 2 drops of geranium essential oil to 1 tablespoon of base oil—this could be almond, grapeseed, or jojoba oil—and mix well.

• Stroking: using the fingertips of both hands, apply the oil to your face, starting with the forehead and moving out to the temples. Repeat the movement. Move on to the nose and move out to the cheeks, and repeat. From the chin, move up the jawline to the ears, and repeat.

• Circling: place your middle and index fingers together between your nose and upper lip and move them in a circular motion around your mouth. Then add your ring fingers to your middle and index fingers and begin applying gentle pressure with a circular movement around your forehead. Start in the middle of your forehead and move out toward the temples. Begin again at the nose and move out to the cheeks. Then begin again at your chin and move up the jawline to the ears.

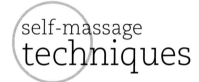

## self-massage techniques

Begin a self-massage by gently stroking the skin, using two hands, alternating the strokes. You can use any of the following techniques.

• rubbing: to stimulate circulation and release muscle tension, rub your muscles in a circular motion with your palms or fingers

• kneading: knead your muscles as if you kneading bread dough

• tapping: use rhythmic knocking or light slapping with the flat of your hand to improve blood circulation and to help relax your muscles

• finish by stroking: when you have completed your massage, end by stroking your skin gently, moving the strokes slowly outward

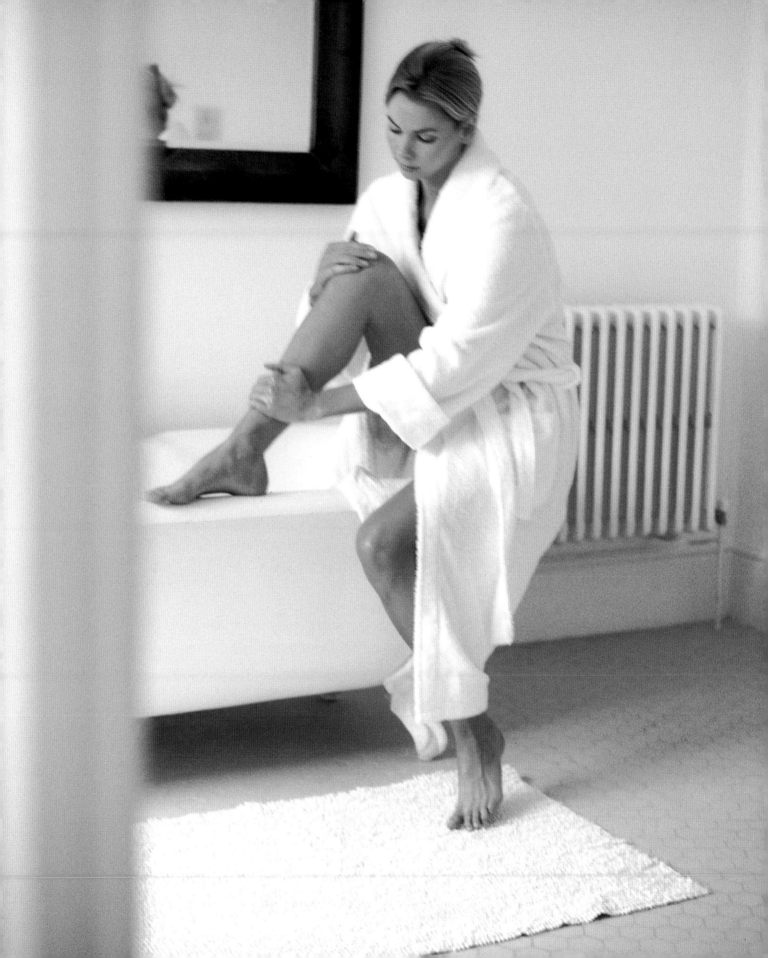

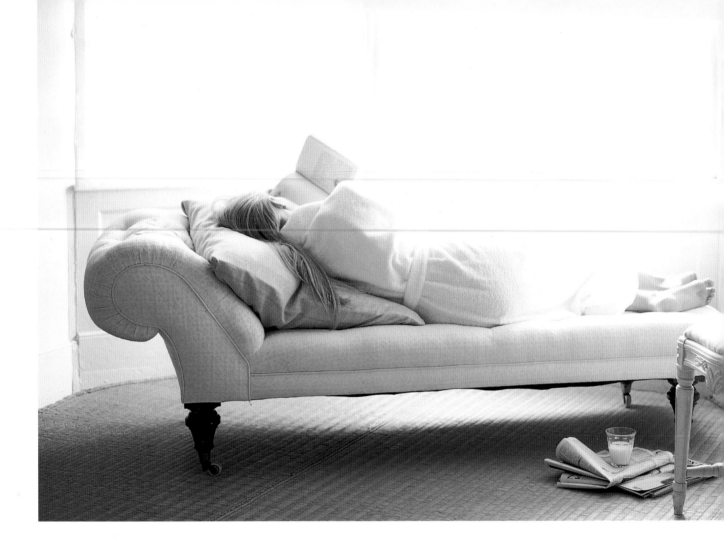

• Patting: to finish, lightly tap your entire face with your index, middle, and ring fingers of both hands. Move from the center of your forehead outward, then from your nose outward, from the top of your lip outward, and from your chin outward.

### detox your stress

Stress and how you deal with it can have a huge impact on your health and wellbeing. When you feel stressed, your skin and hair suffer, and you probably find it hard to sleep, to concentrate, or to stay motivated.

To get the full benefits of detoxing your body, you need to find a way to deal with stress and learn how to give yourself physical and mental breaks from your busy life. Exercise is a wonderful way to let go of physical stress, but sometimes you need to be able to let go and relax instead of being active. When this is the case, a form of meditation could help.

Meditation creates a focused but relaxed mind. Its benefits include improved concentration, increased self-awareness, and an enhanced ability to cope with stress. There are numerous meditation techniques, but all you need is a simple method that suits you. For a start, try the candle meditation described opposite.

### pamper yourself

Demonstrating that you care about yourself is important to establishing and maintaining self-esteem.

When you have completed a detox or even when you have simply cut down on a stress-inducing activity, give yourself a treat. Buy yourself a new outfit, arrange a trip to the hairdresser or a reflexology session, or spend an afternoon watching your favorite video.

Remember that feeling good about yourself is as crucial to your physical wellbeing as doing those things that are good for your body—so don't miss out!

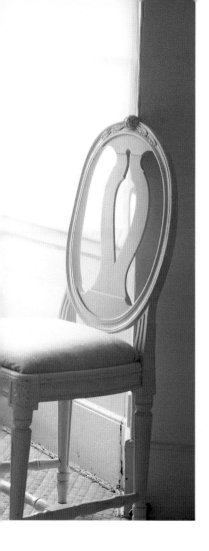

# candle
## meditation

One of the easiest methods of meditation is candle watching. Try it after taking a soothing bath or shortly before going to bed. Allow 10–20 minutes for the meditation.

Sit on the floor or on a chair in a darkened room with a candle lit in front of you at eye level. Breathe in slowly and gently, keeping your eyes on the flame. Try to keep your breathing calm and relaxed. As you stare at the flame, sooner or later thoughts will enter your mind.

When you become aware of a thought, simply let it go and return your attention to the candle flame.

After you have repeated this exercise several times, you should find your mind becoming calm and relaxed.

What you are doing is giving your mind a break and learning how to focus it at will.

When you have finished the meditation, take a deep breath and blow out the candle.

Try not to revert at once to thinking about your troubles. Let yourself feel the benefits of a clear, relaxed mind and then reflect on something positive or go to sleep.

pampering yourself is an effective way to boost your self-esteem

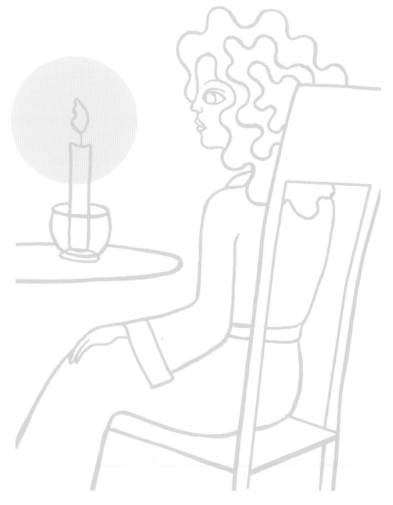

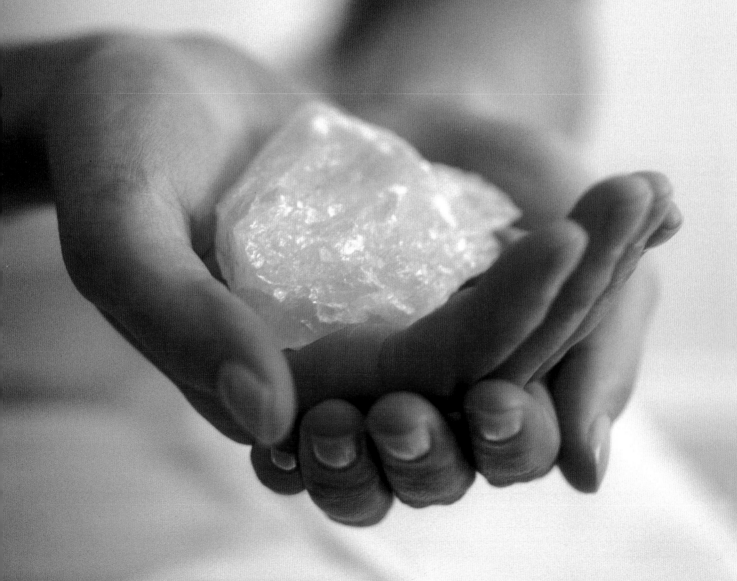

# 5 use the power tools

No two people are the same—so, to achieve optimal
physical, emotional, mental, and spiritual health, you have
to follow your own path. Crystal therapy, aromatherapy,
and herbalism are among the many tools that can help.

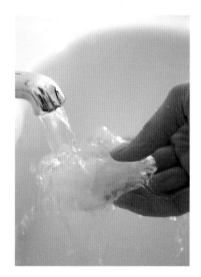

### the healing power of crystals

Crystals have a long history of being valued for both their beauty and their healing properties, and many people still put their faith in crystals, even though—as is the case with many other alternative therapies—the true source of their power remains a mystery.

Crystals can help you to detox your body in various ways, but one of the easiest ways to benefit from their properties is to wear them around your neck or to carry them with you. Many types of crystal pendant are available from crystal or new age shops.

No matter what problem you are trying to resolve, choose the crystal that you are most attached to. Then find out the meaning behind the crystal you chose—you may be surprised at how intuitive you are. If the crystal you have chosen is not on a chain, carry it in a pouch in your pocket or handbag.

### what to do with your crystal

When you have chosen your crystal and brought it home, run it under cold water to cleanse away old energy. If you feel your crystal would benefit from being revitalized, place it outdoors in a sunny position and leave it there for a day.

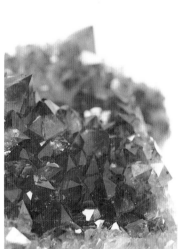

### tune into your crystal

When you have acquired a crystal, you need to decide on its purpose. Relax and hold your crystal with both hands cupped around it. Visualize an energy connection between you and your crystal. This could take the form of a soothing light that surrounds you and the crystal, or a ray of light that comes from your heart to the crystal.

With the purpose of the crystal in mind, say either aloud or to yourself, "Crystal, work with me to help me to … (detox, forgive, be courageous)."

When you have made your request clear, thank the crystal and be confident that it will be helping you to achieve your goal.

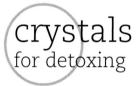

# crystals
## for detoxing

These are the some of the most useful crystals for detoxing:

• **amethyst** cleanses and protects

• **bloodstone** purifies and strengthens

• **celestite** revitalizes and helps in the recalling of dreams

• **citrine** cleanses, dispels fear, and encourages openness

• **clear quartz** aids meditation

• **hermatite** protects and transforms negativity

• **lapis lazuli** boosts mental clarity and protects against depression

• **moonstone** calms the emotions

• **rose quartz** helps to expel excess fluids and impurities

• **tiger's eye** boosts inner strength

# herbs for detoxing

Here is a selection of herbs that will help to detox your body, build your immune system, and relieve stress.

| herb | physical benefits | can be taken as | caution |
|---|---|---|---|
| burdock root | eliminates toxins, clears the skin, balances hormones; a liver tonic | tea, tincture, capsules, tablets | |
| dandelion leaf | helps to relieve urinary tract infections, skin eruptions, stomach pains; purifies the blood; a liver tonic | tea, tincture, capsules, tablets | |
| echinacea | eliminates toxins, purifies the blood, strengthens the immune system | tea, tincture, capsules, tablets | avoid if you have TB, lupus, MS, or autoimmune or collagen diseases |
| evening primrose | improves circulation, regenerates the liver, relieves PMS, reduces cholesterol levels | oil from seeds in capsule form as directed | avoid if you have epilepsy |
| lemon balm | relaxes, improves digestion, relieves irritable bowels, counteracts anxiety and depression | tea; good as an everyday drink | |
| milk thistle | regenerates the liver, counteracts bile stagnation, improves spleen function | tea, tincture, capsules, tablets | |
| nettle | improves function of the small intestine, bladder, and lungs; relieves allergies and asthma | tea, tincture, capsules, tablets | |
| red clover | purifies the blood, nourishes the skin | tea, tincture, capsules, tablets | |
| rosemary | helps clear thinking, improves circulation, boosts nervous system | tea, tincture | |
| sage | improves digestion and bladder function; a natural antiseptic | tea, tincture | avoid in pregnancy or if you have epilepsy |
| sarsaparilla | purifies the blood, improves skin conditions such as eczema and psoriasis; a liver tonic | tea, tincture, capsules, tablets | |
| uva ursi | improves liver, spleen and kidney functions, fights infections; a diuretic | tea, capsules, tablets | |
| vervain | soothes nerves, relieves headaches and depression, aids relaxation | tea, tincture | |
| yarrow | eliminates toxins, encourages sweating, improves digestion, fights infection, counteracts water retention | tea, tincture, capsules, tablets | can cause skin rash; avoid in pregnancy |
| yellow dock | eliminates toxins, clears the skin, improves liver, gall bladder, and bowel functions | tea, tincture, capsules, tablets | |

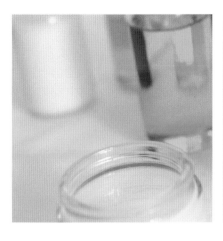
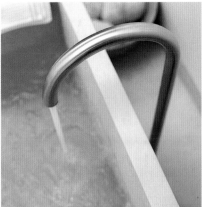
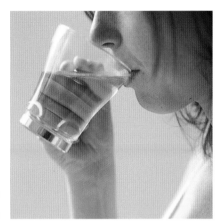

## versatile herbs

The curative power of herbs and their ability to detox the body and promote wellbeing has been recognized for thousands of years.

Herbal remedies can be taken internally to help support the body's own detoxing processes. They are available in many forms, including fresh or dried herbs for tea and herbal supplements in the form of capsules, tablets, powders, and tinctures. Herbs may also be incorporated into creams and oils for external use, and they can be added to bath water or used as poultices.

You can purchase herbs from many health food shops, from special herbal stores, and by mail order. Some herbs can be grown very easily in your garden.

The strength of different herbs and individual sensitivity to various herbs can vary. Some species are very powerful and should be taken with care. If you are concerned that an herb may be too strong, start with a smaller amount than recommended. Herbs should not be used in therapeutic doses for more than 12 weeks, unless recommended by a qualified herbalist. If you are taking any prescribed medication, consult a qualified herbalist before taking herbal remedies.

## making herbal tea

For the purpose of detoxing your body, taking herbs in tea form has a double benefit since you are combining the herbs with water, which also helps to flush out the toxins. For this reason, most of the herbs listed opposite can be made into teas, although there is usually the option of taking them in the form of capsules, tablets, or tinctures. Some herbs can be combined, but to avoid overloading your body, stick to a combination of two or three. If in doubt, seek the advice of a qualified herbalist.

The quantity of herb needed to make a tea varies according to the strength of the herb, but the general rule is to pour a cup of boiling water onto 1 teaspoon of dried herb or 2 teaspoons of fresh herb. Leave to steep for 10 minutes, then remove the herb by straining. Most herbal teas are usually taken as one cup three times a day.

## using a tincture

Tinctures are herbs in liquid form. They are made from herbal extractions steeped in water and alcohol. Drops of the tincture are added to water to be drunk. The usual proportion is between 5 and 15 drops of tincture to half a cup of water—this can be taken two to three times a day. To evaporate most of the traces of alcohol, add your tincture to hot water.

## culinary herbs

Fresh herbs such as basil, chives, coriander, mint, and parsley make excellent additions to salads and soups, and are often used as garnishes. Many fresh herbs contain antioxidants and have specific detoxing effects (see page 47). Rosemary, sage, and thyme are all good detoxing herbs to use during cooking.

### the benefits of aromatherapy

Aromatherapy is the art and science of using essential oils to improve physical, emotional and mental wellbeing. Made from flowers, fruits, and parts of plants, each oil has its own unique properties that can be used to treat conditions affecting the body or the mind.

One of the most beneficial effects of using essential oils comes from the aroma they produce. The aroma has a direct effect on the part of the brain that governs the emotions—which is why each oil has what is called an "emotional profile." Essential oils can also benefit the body by absorption through the skin in massage or by being added to bath water.

### using essential oils with caution

Since the active ingredient in an essential oil is highly concentrated, the oil should always be diluted with a base oil before being applied to the skin. Vegetable oils such as grapeseed or soy are perfect for this purpose. Oils containing vitamin E, such as jojoba and avocado, are sometimes blended with essential oils to make richer skin preparations, especially for dry skin conditions.

To test your skin for sensitivity, dab a small amount of the essential oil that has been diluted in a vegetable oil on the inside of your wrist and leave it overnight; if there is any adverse reaction, do not use that oil.

Children under the age of 18 months should not be treated with essential oils, and no one should take an essential oil internally except on professional advice.

### inhaling, bathing and massage

Here are some of the best ways in which essential oils can be used in a detox program.

• Direct inhalation: simply take the cap off the bottle and breathe in the aroma.

• Steaming: add 5–8 drops of essential oil to a bowl full of hot water; put a towel over your head, lean over the bowl, and gently inhale the steam for about 5 minutes.

• Diffusing: if you have an aromatherapy diffuser, follow the manufacturer's instructions. A diffuser consists of a container to which water and oil are added; the container is then placed over a lit candle and the oil's aromatic vapors are diffused into the air as the water is heated. A general guide is to add 5–10 drops of essential oil to the container full of water.

• Bathing: stir 5–10 drops of essential oil into a full bathtub of water, after the water has finished running; it is better not to use soap with essential oils.

• Massage: make a massage oil by mixing up to 5 drops of an essential oil to every 2 teaspoons of pure vegetable oil such jojoba, grapeseed, or almond oil. The massage oil can be used for either a full massage or a spot massage.

• Air freshening: add 5 drops of an essential oil to every 2 teaspoons of water in a mist spray bottle and shake before spraying.

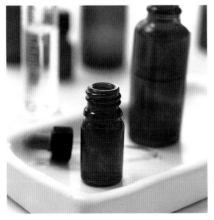
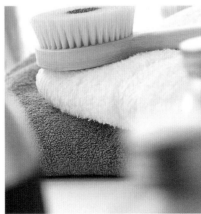
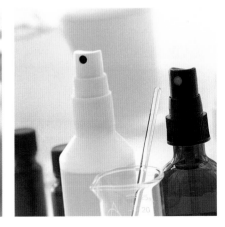

# essential oils for detoxing

Many oils commonly used in aromatherapy can be beneficial in the detoxing process.

| oil | physical benefits | emotional profile | caution |
| --- | --- | --- | --- |
| black pepper | eliminates toxins, boosts circulation, fights infections, energizes | encourages moving on, boosts bravery, endurance | do not use in high doses; could cause irritation |
| cypress | eliminates toxins, stimulates the immune system | relieves stress, grief, self-hate, jealousy, loss, loneliness, regret | avoid if pregnant or if you have high blood pressure, cancer, or fibrosis |
| eucalyptus | relieves asthma, eases aching joints; a decongestant | boosts clear thinking, soothes heated emotions | avoid if you have epilepsy or high blood pressure |
| fennel | eliminates toxins, relieves digestive and menopausal problems | helps to overcome creativity blocks, resistance to change, fear of failure | avoid if pregnant or if you have epilepsy |
| frankincense | helps breathing, rejuvenates mature skin, improves appearance of scars | psychically cleansing, helps to relieve grief, repressed feelings | avoid if pregnant |
| geranium | balances hormones, eases tension and nervous exhaustion, reduces fluid retention | helps to relieve acute fear, heartache, lack of self-esteem, discontentment, | avoid if pregnant |
| grapefruit | detoxifies, stimulates, and energizes; eases muscle fatigue; astringent for oily skin | helps to relieve self-doubt, grief, dependency, frustration | do not use before exposure to sun or sunbeds |
| juniper | purifies, eliminates toxins, improves mental clarity, reduces fluid retention, energizes | helps to relieve guilt, discontentment, defensive behaviour | avoid if pregnant or if you have kidney disease |
| lavender | eases tension headaches, helps breathing, lowers high blood pressure, promotes sleep | helps to relieve insecurity, trauma, fear, addiction, obsessive behavior | |
| lemon | eliminates toxins, reduces cellulite, balances nervous system | helps to relieve resentment, distrust, irrational thinking, apathy | may irritate sensitive skin; do not use before exposure to sun |
| orange (sweet) | relieves stress, reduces cellulite | helps to relieve apathy, worry, addiction, lethargy, depression | do not use before exposure to sun or sunbeds |
| peppermint | reduces pain, helps breathing, improves mental clarity and memory | helps to lift mood, relieves shock, apathy, helplessness | use with caution; may irritate sensitive skin; avoid if pregnant |
| pine | helps breathing, relieves muscle and joint aches, boosts immunity, energizes | helps to transform feelings of inadequacy, regret, self-blame | avoid if you have prostate cancer |
| sandalwood | heals skin, reduces stress, helps breathing, promotes restful sleep | helps to relieve insecurity, loneliness, nightmares, dwelling on the past | |
| ylang ylang | relaxes tense muscles, promotes restful sleep, lowers high blood pressure | helps to relieve anxiety, resentment, jealousy, frustration, anger, irritability | |

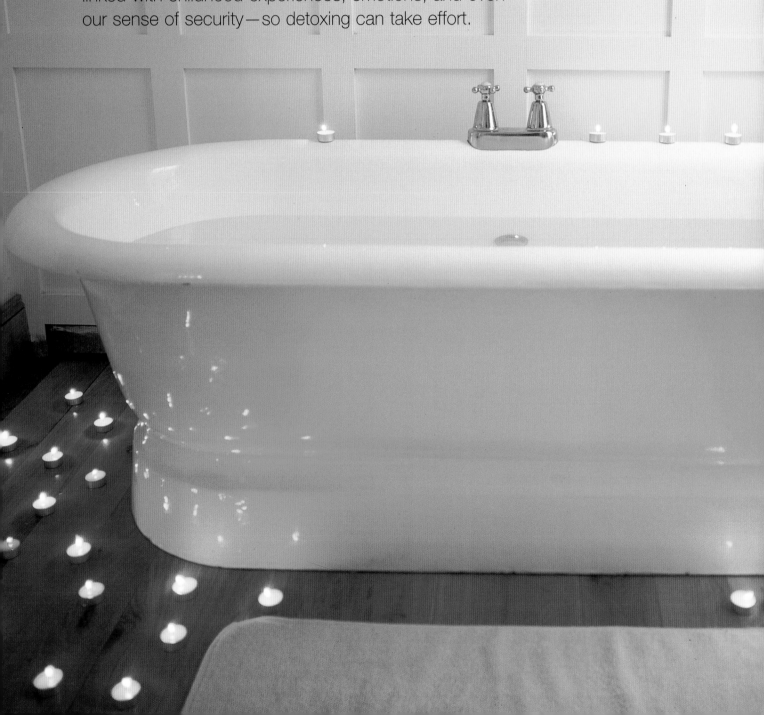

# do it now

Purifying the body is about banishing toxins that have built up over time and changing physical habits to create a healthier lifestyle. Those habits may be closely linked with childhood experiences, emotions, and even our sense of security—so detoxing can take effort.

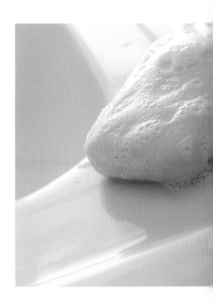

### gentleness and patience

There is no need to be cruel to your body by overdoing toxic treats one minute and withholding them the next. You are far more likely to have positive and lasting results from a detox program if you are kind to your body and do what is right for you.

Whatever approach you take to a physical detox, it is important to give your body time to expel toxins and to monitor the effects of the detox. You may decide to do this over a period of a week or a month, but if you notice any persistent ill-effects, such as dizziness or lethargy, stop the regime and seek the advice of your doctor.

### troubleshooting

*I find it hard to follow a detox diet even for two days*
Don't chastize yourself if you find it too difficult to stick to a detox diet. Maybe now is not the best time to be doing it. Let it go and try again when you're ready. Even partially following the diet will bring some benefits.

*I find it hard to keep up the exercises*
You'll find it easier to follow an exercise regime if it's simple and can fit into your routine with ease. If you allocate specific time to your exercises and do them without fail, however you're feeling, you'll find that they become just another habit like brushing your teeth.

*I've tried the tips and I still find it hard to fall asleep*
There are many non-addictive herbal sleeping tablets available from pharmacies and health food stores. If you can also find a suitable guided meditation tape, the combination can be very effective.

*I find it difficult to relax completely*
Relaxation has a lot to do with letting go, and like any other skill, it takes practice. If you find that you really cannot let go of your problems and yet you cannot come up with any solutions, it may be advisable to seek professional help.

*I don't feel that I deserve to be pampered*
Everyone deserves to be pampered or given a treat from time to time. It will boost your self-esteem and make you feel good.

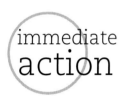

## immediate action

Over the next 24 hours, think about what you could do to start detoxing your body. You could cut down on the amount of caffeine or chocolate you consume, for example. You could begin a new exercise regime or rid yourself of stress by having a soothing bath followed by a calming meditation. Choose one or more of the detox tools presented in this chapter and incorporate it into your life today.

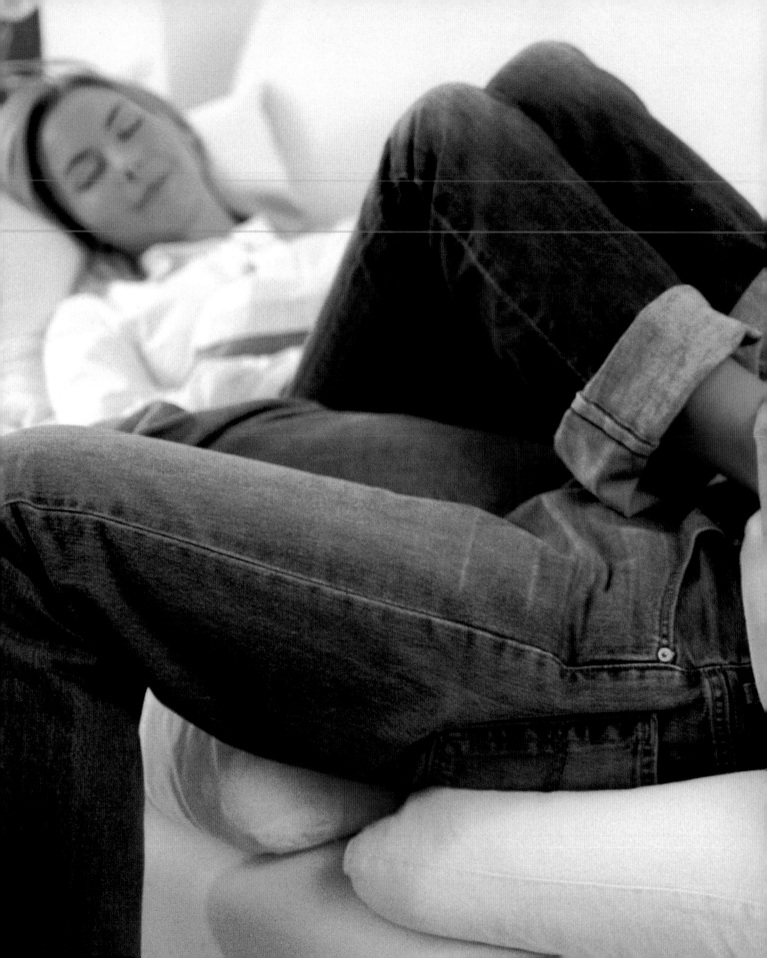

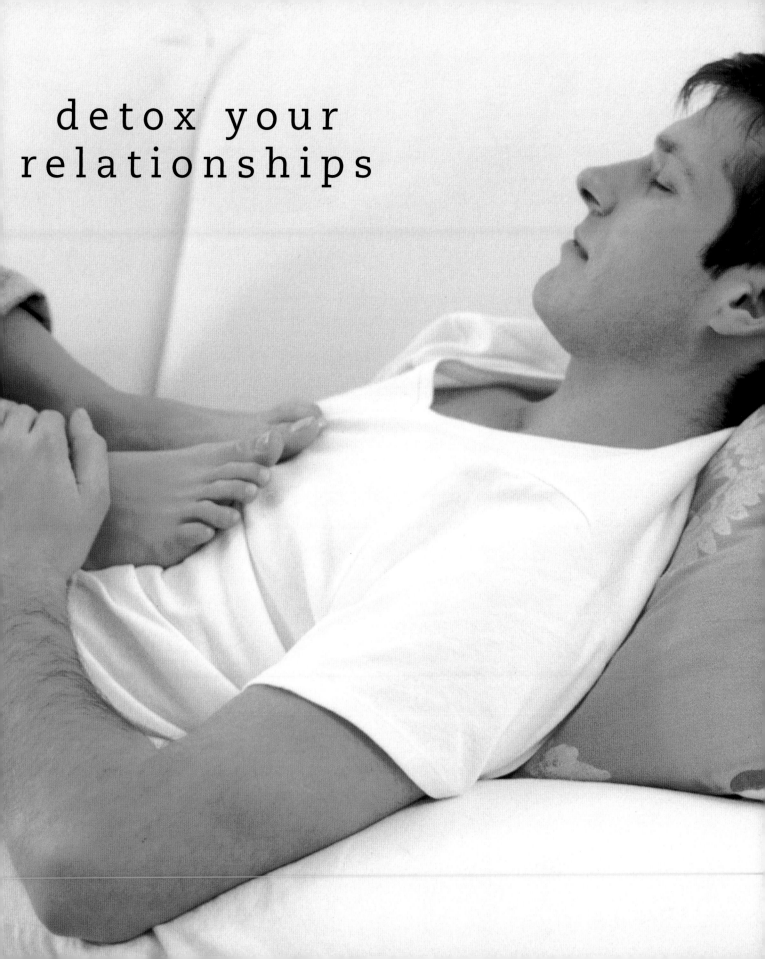

detox your
relationships

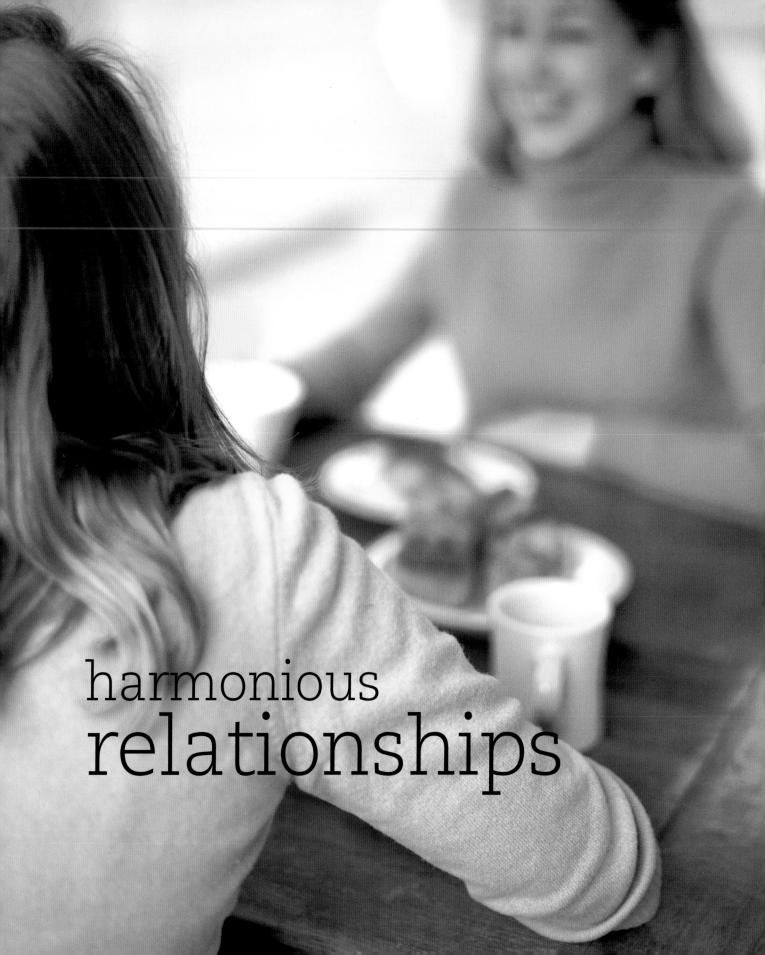

harmonious
relationships

Whether they involve lovers, friends, colleagues, or family members, relationships can have a powerful impact on all aspects of our lives, particularly our happiness and the way we feel about ourselves.

When relationships work well, they can give us a sense of belonging as well as opportunities to grow, to have fun, and to make sense of the world. Relationships that don't work well can be detrimental to our health and well-being. They can drain our time, our energy, and sometimes our resources, and may even encourage us to make the wrong choices.

This chapter is about freeing yourself from people who affect your life negatively, so that you can focus on relationships that are truly beneficial. When you start reading it, remember that all relationships involve a two-way exchange, and even though your new behavior may lead others to respond differently, the only person you can really change is yourself.

Following the four steps to detoxing your relationships will help you understand yourself and others better, teach you to spot real and false friendships, and give you the tools to transform or let go of those relationships that no longer serve you.

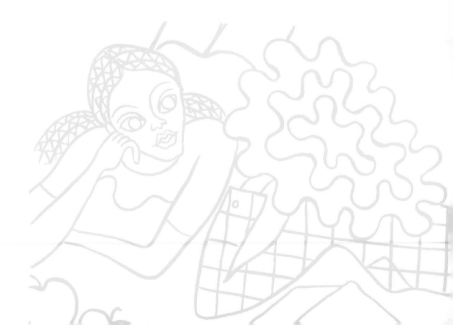

# 1 know who you are

Achieving a more profound understanding of yourself and the people around you is the first step to setting up a framework for detoxing your relationships.

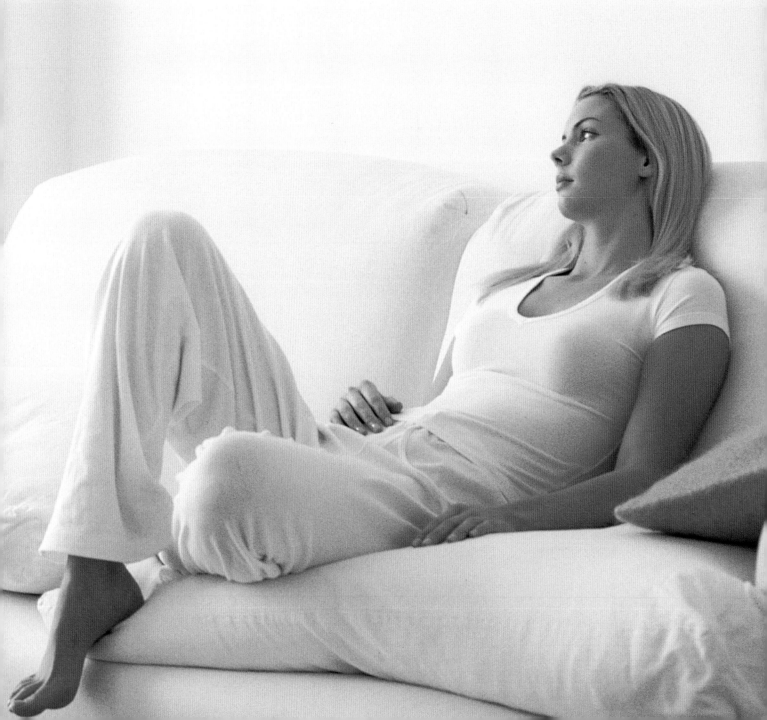

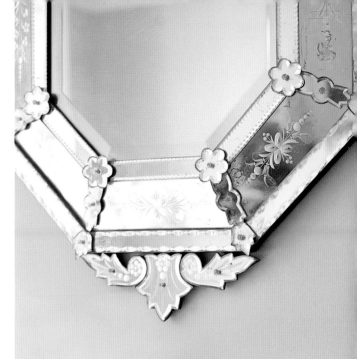

## analyzing your personality

One of the simplest and most revealing methods of personality analysis is the enneagram, an ancient system that is still used by psychologists today. It is founded on the theory that there are nine personality types (see right) and—while each of us has a mixture of all nine personalities in our character—one personality type dominates in each individual. The dominant type is usually adopted in childhood in response to childhood relationships and experiences.

If you are not sure which personality type you are, turn the page and read the four statements below the name of each type to see which one describes your character most accurately. If you can't make up your mind, get a close friend or family member to help.

The nine types are also divided into three groups according to the way they perceive life.

• The feeling group—Helper, Achiever, Individualist—experiences life through feelings. The Helper's feelings are linked to helping others. The Achiever's feelings are linked to achieving goals, and the Individualist's feelings are linked to creative expression.

• The thinking group—Thinker, Loyalist, Enthusiast—experiences life through thought. The Thinker is intensely analytical. The Loyalist's thinking is directed by the desire to improve standards, while the Enthusiast focuses on keeping mentally occupied.

• The instinctive group—Perfectionist, Leader, Mediator—experiences life through their instincts. Perfectionists use their instincts to strive for perfection. Leaders act instinctively to achieve their goals. Mediators use their instincts to create a harmonious environment.

## nine types of personality

• the Perfectionist is organized, idealistic, and intolerant

• the Helper is caring, helpful, and manipulative

• the Achiever is self-assured, ambitious, and hostile

• the Individualist is creative, emotional, and depressive

• the Thinker is intellectual, analytical, and eccentric

• the Loyalist is courageous, responsible, and dependent

• the Enthusiast is excitable, uninhibited, and excessive

• the Leader is assertive, powerful, and destructive

• the Mediator is orderly, principled, and independent

# discover your type

Don't feel that your personality type is fixed and permanent. Most of us behave slightly differently when we are with different people. Insights into your personality type will allow you to achieve a better balance in yourself and in your relationships.

### the perfectionist

- I am critical of myself and others.
- I like to make lists of things I have to do.
- I hate being interrupted in the middle of a task.
- I would like to be more laid back and easy-going.

*If this is you* From an early age, as a result of continual criticism, you learned to control yourself and to take responsibility for your actions. As a result, you have a tough inner critic that makes you constantly strive to improve everything you do. You can be an energetic, considerate, and inspiring leader, but your high standards make it likely that you have a pessimistic streak.

*Relating to others* You are self-controlled and secretive, preferring to keep your personal feelings and opinions to yourself, but once you take on a relationship, you are loyal, caring, and often keep your friends for life.

*Staying balanced* You would be happier in yourself if you were willing to share more time with other people and concentrate on becoming more relaxed and less rigid in your ideas about right and wrong.

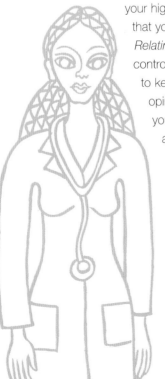

### the helper

- I find it hard to say no when people ask for my help.
- I sometimes find it difficult to see things through.
- I prefer working with people than with machines, ideas, or figures.
- I enjoy helping others to achieve their goals.

*If this is you* As a child, you felt your survival depended on the approval of others and, as a result, you learned to earn love through meeting other people's needs. You are caring and compassionate, which makes you a warm-hearted friend, although you can be domineering and manipulative when you want to have your own way.

*Relating to others* You adapt your feelings to make others feel good. You are committed to helping those you love and often give more than you receive. This concentration on others can make you feel as if nobody knows the real you.

*Staying balanced* Think more about your own needs and encourage relationships in which you allow others to give you as much as you give them.

### the achiever

- I feel positive when I am with other people but depressed when I am alone.
- I never let myself get too dependent on others.
- Without goals to work toward, I get bored and lethargic.
- I find it difficult to relax and do nothing.

*If this is you* As a child, you were loved and rewarded for your achievements, and as a result, you learned to suspend your own desires in favor of achieving the success that guaranteed that you would continue to be loved. Your self-assurance and ability to entertain makes you popular, but you can become vindictive and dishonest if you feel threatened.

*Relating to others* You are adaptable and make people laugh, but a fear of rejection means that you tend to hide your deeper feelings; this sometimes makes you appear uncaring, aggressive, and abrupt.

*Staying balanced* You should allow yourself to become more vulnerable by expressing your true feelings and concerns to those around you.

### the individualist

• I like to be seen as an individual and am attracted to unusual things.
• I spend time wondering about the meaning of my life.
• I appreciate nature, beauty, and creativity.
• I feel a kaleidoscope of emotions.

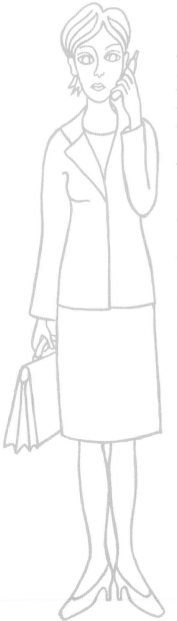

each person's character is made up of a mixture of all nine types of personality

*If this is you* At some point during your childhood, you felt abandoned and alone. As a result, you still suffer from the feeling of something missing in your life. You are creative and introspective, and more likely to express your emotions through your work than by confiding in other people. When you fail to achieve your goals, you can develop self-destructive feelings.

*Relating to others* You are compassionate and sensitive. Although you like to be understood, you often hold yourself back through fear of responsibility. You may feel that no one really knows you well.

*Staying balanced* Try to become less self-conscious and fearful by using your natural sensitivity and understanding to focus your attention on others.

### the thinker

• I like to be alone to ponder on and sort out difficult problems in life.
• I have a constant thirst for new knowledge and adventure.
• I often hold a different point of view from others.
• Personal freedom, space, and individualism are very important to me.

*If this is you* As a child, you felt that your freedom and privacy were intruded on by others, and as a result, you became emotionally distant, withdrawing into a world of the mind.

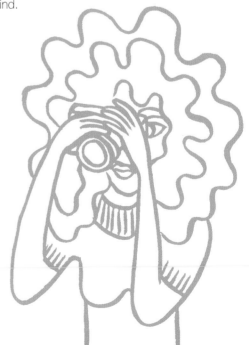

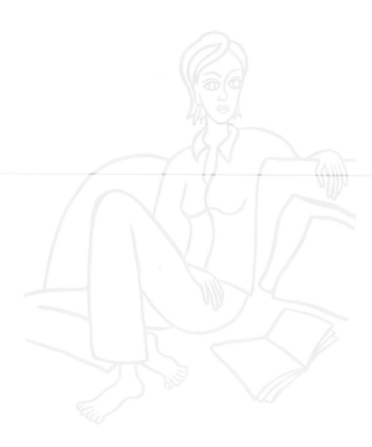

*If this is you* As a child, you felt let down by authority figures, which left you feeling suspicious about other people's motives. As a result, you tend either to look for someone protective or to reject authority altogether. You can be courageous and warm-hearted, but when you feel insecure, you can become anxious and dependent.

*Relating to others* Loyal and generous, you have a genuine interest in the welfare of others and are willing to work hard to improve the standard of living for everyone. Team work is important, and you need to feel a sense of belonging.

*Staying balanced* You should learn how to exercise your inner authority to help yourself and others feel supported and secure.

## the enthusiast

- I find it easy to come up with solutions for other people's problems.
- I like to be flexible and tend to avoid making too many long-term plans.
- I can hold a conversation with almost anyone.
- I get bored easily and enjoy mental challenges.

*If this is you* As a child, you learned to avoid uncomfortable feelings by escaping into your imagination. As a result, you often refuse to acknowledge difficulties, preferring to concentrate on something more exciting. Your many interests give you great potential, but you may be too busy having fun to become deeply involved in anything long term.

*Relating to others* You are seen as a source of adventure and excitement, but you can be offensive when pursuing something important. You value those closest to you, but often ignore problems that need to be resolved.

*Staying balanced* You need to take more responsibility for your emotions by dealing with difficult and painful feelings in yourself and others.

Independent and intelligent, you enjoy having time alone to think, and your extraordinary powers of perception give you the ability to formulate original and inventive ideas.

*Relating to others* You tend to become attached to a few specially chosen people who share your interests and respect your privacy and freedom. You may find social attachments hard work, giving you a reputation for being strange and eccentric.

*Staying balanced* Be open to increasing the range of your relationships, try to learn more about other people by spending time with them and sharing the knowledge that you have acquired.

## the loyalist

- I like to keep busy with a full schedule.
- My home, family, and relationships are my priority.
- I take responsibility seriously and hate irresponsibility in others.
- I work hard and like to be organized.

### the leader

- I have clear ideas about what is right and wrong.
- It annoys me when people don't get to the point directly.
- I find being in charge easy and enjoyable.
- I often find disagreements exhilarating.

*If this is you* As a child, your experiences led you to believe that only strong people were respected. As a result, you learned to protect yourself by being assertive and taking control. On the positive side,

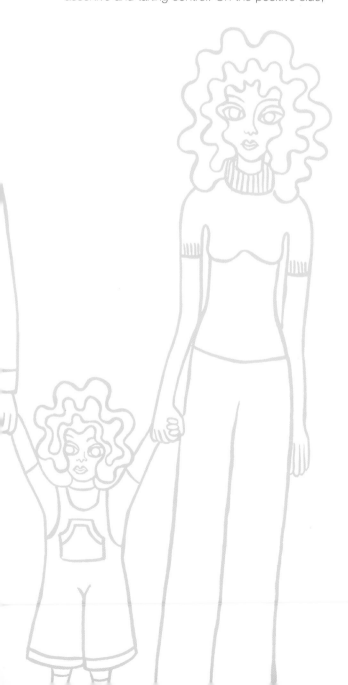

you can be fair and courageous, sticking up for those who are more vulnerable than you. On the negative side, you can be ruthless and hardhearted.

*Relating to others* You are fiercely loyal and protective in your relationships with others. You are very close to your family, and your home is often the only place where you feel relaxed enough to be caring and loving without feeling threatened.

*Staying balanced* You need to have more compassion for others, taking into account their feelings, needs, and concerns in relation to your goals.

### the mediator

- I am regarded by most people as someone who has plenty of common sense.
- I dislike arguments and usually try to avoid them.
- I am independent, and my opinions are not easily swayed by others.
- I think that people often create their own difficulties in life.

*If this is you* As a child, you were given reason to believe that your needs and feelings were repeatedly overlooked. As a result, you learned to forget about yourself and turn your attention to other things and other people's concerns. You tend to be easygoing and accommodating. You dislike dealing with problems and volatile emotions, preferring to keep the peace even if it means being obstinate.

*Relating to others* You are kind, compassionate, and dependable. You are cautious of others, but once you get to know someone you make a trustworthy friend. You like to be a part of a group, working toward achieving a worthwhile cause.

*Staying balanced* You need to make sure that you stand up for yourself, recognize your own importance, and express your values and feelings openly.

# 2 know how you are seen

Most people make up their minds how they feel about you in the first four minutes of contact. If you project a poor image, you could reduce your opportunities by hiding your true qualities, so take time to consider how you come across.

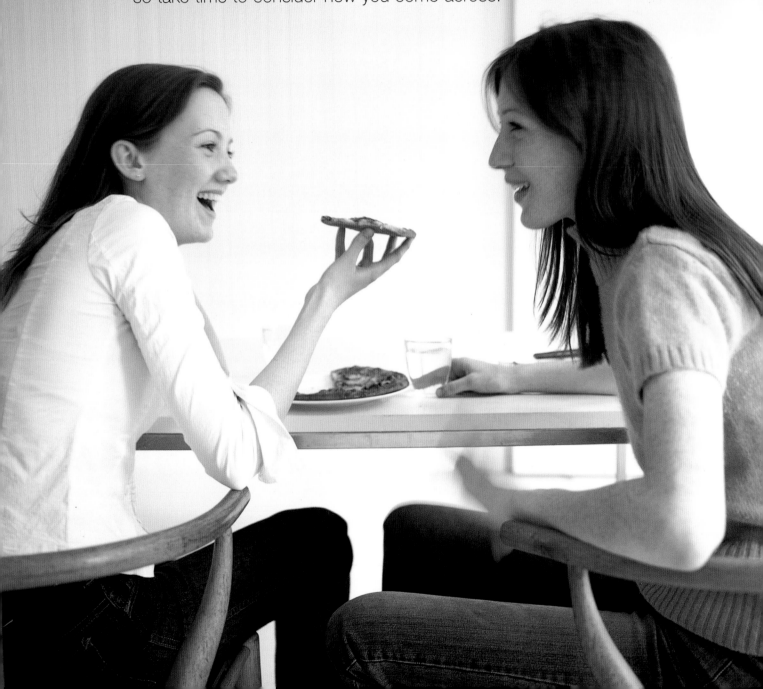

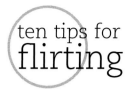

# ten tips for flirting

If you want to flirt successfully with someone, you should:

• smile a lot

• laugh a lot

• hold the other person's gaze for slightly longer than usual

• give a sideways glance over slightly raised shoulders

• run your fingers through your hair

• expose your wrists

• stand or sit close to the other person

• touch the other person's arms or legs

• lean toward the other person

• cross your legs toward the other person

improving your image will allow you to make the most of your good qualities

## the power of body language

One obvious area to address when it comes to improving your image is body language. The way you hold your body, your facial expressions, your hand gestures, and the amount of eye contact you give can reveal more about what you are feeling and thinking than the words you speak. Here are ten impressions to avoid if you want to project a positive image and the body language associated with them.

*Bossiness*
Using hand gestures with palms facing down.

*Nervousness*
Fiddling with your hair, buttons, or any other small object.

*Dishonesty*
Putting a hand over your face or mouth when talking.

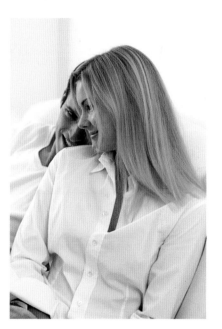

*Dominance*
Staring at the person you are talking to for longer than normal.

*Superiority*
Holding your head back and looking down your nose at the person you are talking to.

*Stubbornness*
Holding onto your knee or leg when sitting down.

*Self-control*
Crossing your ankles.

*Criticism*
Holding one arm across your body and one hand on your chin.

*Frustration*
Clasping your hands in front of you; the higher you hold your hands, the more frustrated you appear.

*Ridicule*
Holding your thumbs inside your fists.

# colors for
## healing

- if you are feeling tired, rejected, or lacking in courage, wear red

- if you are feeling angry, frustrated, or need healing, wear green

- if you are feeling melancholy or lethargic, wear orange

- if you are feeling unloved or troubled, wear pink

- if you are feeling stressed or emotional, wear violet

- if you are feeling nervous, indecisive, or tense, wear blue

- if you are feeling depressed, frustrated, or lonely, wear yellow

- if you are feeling oversensitive and vulnerable, wear black

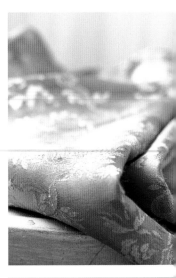

## what color says about you

One of the most important and basic elements in our lives is color. Colors are everywhere: the colors we wear, the colors we paint our walls, the colors we see every day on the way to work, at the office, in the street. The colors we choose to have around us, consciously or subconsciously, project an image to the world. And other people respond to that image—whether we are aware of it or not.

Colors can also be used to alter your mood and the way you are perceived. For example, if you tend to wear predominantly blue or black clothes, try wearing red or pink to see if it affects your feelings, or influences how others see you.

## making a good impression

The use of color is just one way to influence how you are perceived. There are many other ways to improve the impression you give.

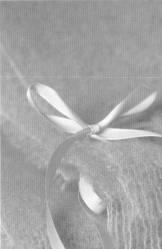

- Dress to suit the occasion; even when you want to look casual, you should be well presented.

- Act as if you are relaxed and comfortable being you.

- Stand or sit with a straight back; hunched or rounded shoulders are a sign of low self-esteem.

- Face the person you are talking to straight on; this will make you appear more confident.

- Use plenty of eye contact and nod every now and then; this shows that you are focused on the person you are talking to and interested in the conversation.

- Smile frequently to show that you are happy to be in another person's company; if you want to appear more reserved, don't show your teeth when you smile.

- Keep your chin up; this conveys a sense of confidence and self-respect.

- Tip your head to one side to show you are listening.

- Keep your gestures open and relaxed; don't cross your arms or put your hands in your pockets.

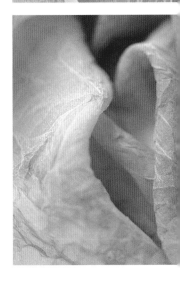

# your color vibration

Like body language, color has a power all of its own. By wearing colors that are best suited to your body and personality, you will not only make a greater impact on those around you, but you will also feel more in control. Color can be useful as a tool for self-knowledge, too. Most people have a strong preference for a particular color, and that color represents their most obvious character traits. Below is a table of eight colors and the personalities they represent. If you don't already have a favorite color, study the list below and see which one you are most attracted to. Then study your chosen color and find out what it says about you.

| color | your charm | your challenge |
|---|---|---|
| red | you have a warm, friendly personality and your assertive, daredevil nature makes you exciting to be with | stubborn, insensitive, and sometimes coarse, you show your irritation by throwing temper tantrums |
| green | adaptable, cooperative, and generous, you make a good listener and prefer life to be harmonious | you sometimes suffer from feelings of inadequacy and may have a demanding or jealous streak |
| orange | enthusiastic, confident, and sociable, you have a restless nature, but are usually happy and buoyant; people like to be with you because of your uplifting and lively presence | you have a tendency to go to extremes, and your restlessness sometimes leads to explosive outbursts of temper |
| pink | affectionate and loving, you treat others with compassion and kindness, and like to be thought of as approachable | when you feel insecure, you can become difficult, dominating, and inconsiderate to those around you |
| violet | although reserved, you like to be an individual, and your natural sensitivity draws others to you | when angry or frustrated, you can be quarrelsome, inconsiderate, and vain |
| blue | you are loyal, conservative, and introspective; people tend to trust you because of your sensitive, sympathetic nature | when you lose interest in something, you become bored and lazy, and find it difficult to concentrate |
| yellow | intelligent and lively, you enjoy being the center of attention; you make a good friend and a loyal confidant | you get frustrated easily, and problems make you nervous, irritable, and short-tempered with others |
| black | disciplined, independent, strong-willed, and rebellious, you like to be in control of your decisions | you can be negative and gloomy, with a tendency to blot out problems without dealing with them |

# 3 value people

Learning to assess the underlying strengths
and weaknesses of your relationships, and
understanding what you want from them,
is the next step on the road to detoxing.

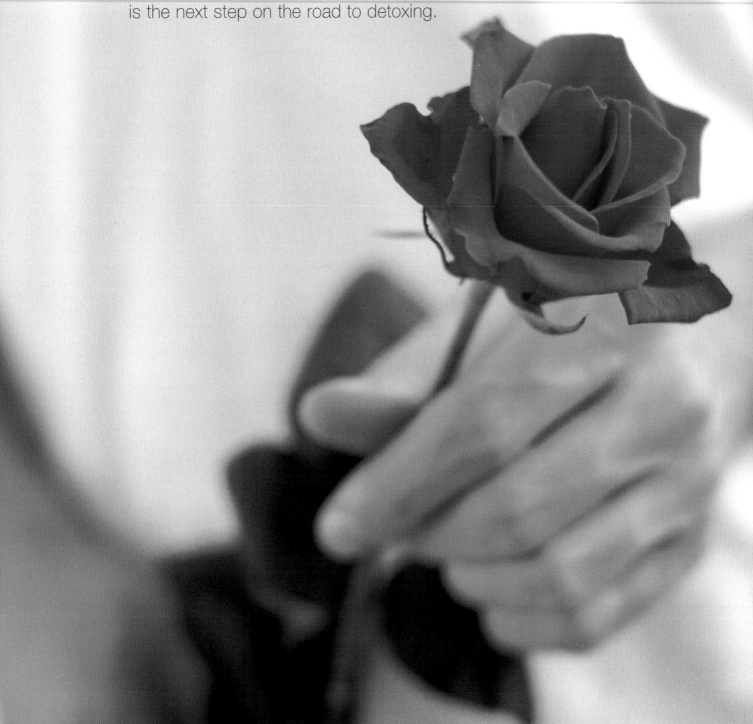

# recognizing a true friend

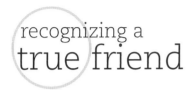

If you want to know whether your friend is a true friend, ask yourself the following questions:

- is this a worthwhile relationship?

- do I feel bad about myself after I've been with this person?

- do I have to censor my opinions?

- is there a fair amount of giving and taking between us?

- could I turn to this person in a crisis?

- is this person genuinely happy when I succeed?

- does this person offer positive support and advice?

- does this person understand me?

## the importance of relationships

When it comes to good health and success, our close relationships can have a positive bearing on all aspects of our lives, from our careers to the way we bring up our children. Recent studies have shown that when people have positive relationships, they endure less stress, recover more quickly from illness, and live longer.

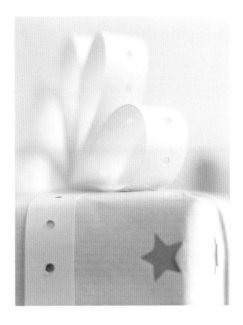

There are some relationships, however, that masquerade as beneficial but in truth are detrimental to our wellbeing. These are the people who often drain our energy and damage our self-esteem. They may be critical when they should be supportive, put us down with veiled insults and sly remarks, or manipulate us to suit their own agenda.

Negative, destructive relationships can be bad for us in many ways, leading to feelings of stress and self-sabotage. However, toxic types are not always easy to spot, especially if we are not looking for them. In fact, some relationships appear to be functioning well when in reality they are doing just the opposite.

## what do you want from a friendship?

As a starting point to identifying toxic people in your life, you need to be clear in your own mind about what you want from a relationship. Most good relationships are based on mutual understanding, reciprocal appreciation, and support for one another. Shared experience is another key quality, which is why you may feel closer to someone you work with or who has had a similar life experience. Sadly, this type of relationship does not always last and may fizzle out if your lives move on and you no longer have anything in common.

To decide what you value, think about someone who is close to you. Write down all the characteristics of that person that makes your relationship successful. When you have finished, add to the list anything else you can think of that you would appreciate in a relationship.

# characterizing a toxic type

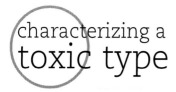

- the Criticizer likes to put you down and make you feel inferior

- the Dominator must be in charge and hates having opinions criticized

- the Insulter pretends to be on your side but makes veiled insults

- the User wants something that you've got, but leaves as soon as something better comes along

- the Whiner divulges problems but is not interested in solutions

- the Competitor always wants to be better than you

- the Manipulator is happy as long as you do what you are told

- the Game Player loves to stir up problems between you and others

- the Discloser enjoys making you squirm by disclosing your secrets

- the Betrayer strings you along and betrays you in a hurtful way

## toxic relationships

There are many types of potentially toxic relationships, and some of them are fairly easy to spot once you know the signs. If you are having a relationship with one of the toxic types listed on the left, you need to think seriously about how beneficial your relationship is.

There are times when it is still possible to save a relationship and times when it is right to end it. Some relationships that only verge on the toxic may be worth repairing, but if you are continually feeling uncomfortable, bad about yourself, angry or crushed when you relate to somebody, it is time to let the relationship go. It may

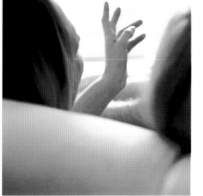

be difficult to admit that a friendship isn't working out, but holding onto a toxic friend may do more harm than good.

Both men and women can find it hard to end a relationship, but women are more likely to want to discuss and analyze what has happened. Men may be content simply to accept that something has gone wrong and walk away without discussion.

## letting go

If you have taken a good, hard look at your relationship and decided that it is not worth saving, it is usually advisable to let go in a gradual way. One option is to tell the other person outright that you no longer want your relationship to continue, and in cases when the person is your lover or partner, a heart-to-heart conversation may be needed to bring the relationship to an end. But in other circumstances, it may be better to wind down the relationship slowly, maybe seeing the other person less frequently, until the relationship fades out. This will help the other person get the hint and resume other relationships.

While honesty is a good policy, there is no point being hurtful, judgmental, or blunt for the sake of it. There may be relationships in your life that are not right for you now, but you may wish to resume them at a later date, so it makes sense, if you can, to bring them to an end in a positive way.

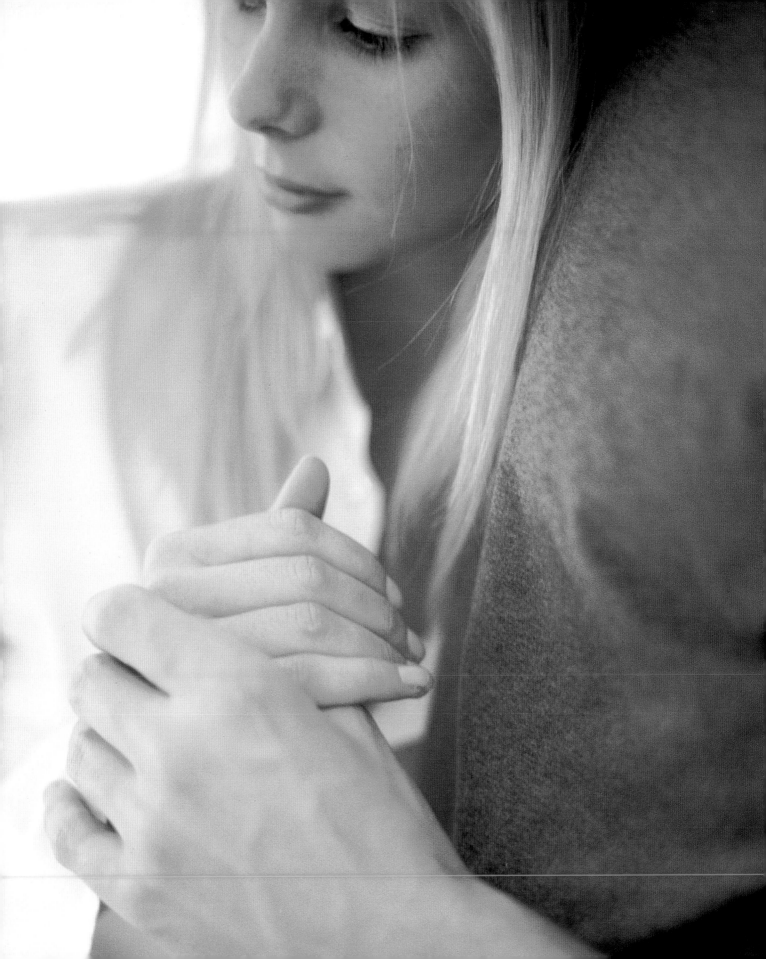

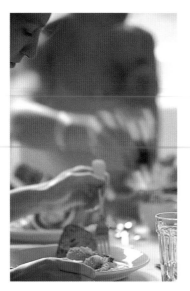

### resolving a toxic relationship

Whether the toxic person in your life is a partner or a friend, if you go about resolving the situation in a methodical way, it will help you to clarify your thoughts and decide whether you want to save and transform the relationship or to cut the ties.

Start by figuring out what makes the other person toxic in your life—for example, does he or she leave you feeling depressed or bad about yourself, give you bad advice on purpose, or drop you in a mess? Think of examples of occasions when the person has behaved in a way that has been toxic to you. Then decide whether you think the relationship is worth saving or whether you want to end it. To help you to make up your mind, try asking yourself the following questions:

*Is the problem that exists between us easily resolved?*
The solution may be as simple as voicing your opinion about something.

*Does this person behave in a toxic way often?*
Remember that everybody has their off days.

*Do I want to invest the time and energy to improve this relationship?*
Sometimes it is worth keeping a relationship on a positive footing if you have to live or work with the person concerned, but at the same time you can become less involved.

*Do I think this person will want to invest the time and energy needed to improve this relationship?*
Be aware that some people, even when they are in the wrong or share half the blame, will decide not to acknowledge or accept their share of the problem.

### putting your cards on the table

If you decide to have it out with the person concerned, approach the situation in a sensitive way. On the down side, communicating your feelings could make the situation worse, if the person feels that you are being

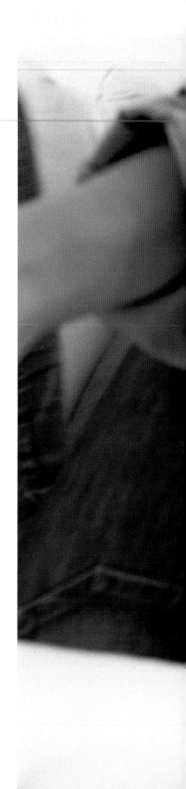

# bad habits
## in a relationship

If your relationship is not working well, the reason could be that you or the other person is exhibiting one or more of the following habits:

• being excessively critical or judgmental about the other person's behavior or interests

• showing a lack of support or respect for the other person's desires and needs.

• being dishonest and censoring your feelings or opinions to fit in with the other person

• giving too much or taking too much

• feeling threatened or jealous of the other persons success and giving misleading advice

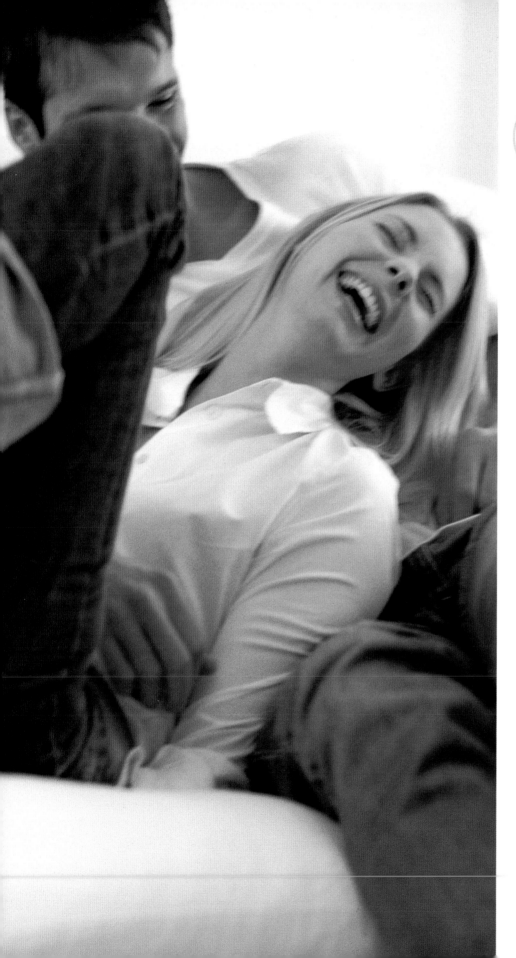

# good aims
## in a relationship

If you want a relationship to succeed, aim to integrate these habits into your life together:

• make time to be together and enjoy each other's company

• show understanding and empathy—genuine relationships thrive on mutual care and respect for each other's desires and needs

• allow the other person freedom to make up his or her own mind, but offer helpful advice and support when needed

• deal with annoyances quickly and honestly, and apologize when necessary; you don't have to agree about everything—sometimes it may be worth agreeing to disagree

• recognize and celebrate each other's successes and encourage each other to achieve more

# detoxing a friendship

**Here are some tips for success when trying to resolve a problem with a friend or partner:**

- **pinpoint what it is that upsets you about the way your friend or partner behaves**

- **bring the subject to the other person's attention in a gentle way, avoiding blame or accusation**

- **listen carefully to what the other person has to say**

- **validate the relationship and express your desire to work through the problem**

- **end your conversation on a positive note**

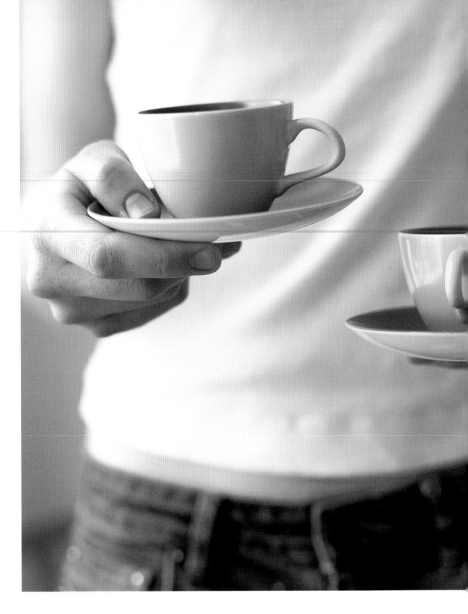

unfair, or blaming or criticizing them; even if what you say is true, it may provoke a defensive reaction, leading to more conflict. Listening carefully, agreeing to disagree, validating the relationship, or saying sorry when appropriate should help to resolve the problem. On the positive side, voicing your grievance could clear the air and bring you closer together.

Alternatively, if you want to let the person concerned know what you feel but don't want to suffer the aftermath of communicating it, write it down on a piece of paper which you can tear up or destroy afterward. There is something very detoxing about putting your thoughts and feelings down on paper. It gives you the opportunity to get what you think and feel out of your system, so that you can let it go.

If you have decided that the relationship is not worth saving or you have tried to improve your relationship but it hasn't worked, it is time to cut the ties. Unless

you like dramatic endings, the best way to do this is to let the person gradually drift out of your life. You can do this by becoming less available, by altering your routine, or by taking up a new interest.

## support yourself in your decision

If you have decided to end the relationship and you have gone about it in the most compassionate way, don't feel guilty. On the other hand, if you have decided to maintain the relationship and you have smoothed over the difficulties between you, don't bother dwelling on it. It takes two people to make a relationship, whether it is a love partnership or a friendship, and it will require give and take from both of you to make it a success.

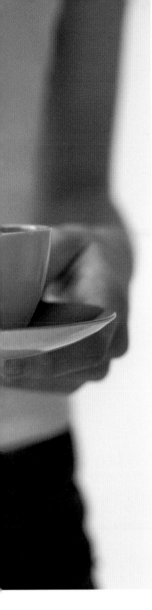

# meditation for harmony

If you have made up your mind to continue your friendship or love partnership, this meditation will help you to let go of negative feelings. It will also harmonize and uplift the connection between you and your friend or partner.

Find a quiet time and a place where you won't be disturbed. Take a few deep breaths, and as you breathe out, release any tension you feel.

Imagine yourself being bathed in a beautiful, warm, soothing light. As the light envelops your body, feel yourself relaxing and letting go of all the things that have been troubling you. Imagine yourself surrounded by a sense of harmony.

Now imagine the person with whom you want to create harmony standing opposite you. Increase the light that surrounds you until it encompasses the other person, too.

Are there any negative feelings or issues that come up when you look at this person—irritation or frustration, for example? If so, imagine them being dissolved in the light, getting smaller and smaller until they disappear.

Say to the other person, "I am letting go of any negative connection between us."

Then think about the gifts your friend or partner brings to the relationship—understanding, humor, love, or other qualities.

Say to the person, "I appreciate and thank you for the gifts you bring to our relationship."

Then think about the gifts you bring and say, "I bring these gifts to the relationship with love."

Imagine the two of you feeling a sense of mutual appreciation and love. Imagine shaking your friend or partner by the hand and hugging or nodding to each other in recognition of your shared understanding.

Let the image of this person go and say to yourself, "I feel good. I have communicated love and appreciation to this person."

Take a few deep breaths, and as you breathe out feel your presence in your body. Open your eyes.

This meditation can work wonders to bring about positive results at a deep level. But bear in mind that each individual has free will, so it will be up to your friend or partner to accept the gifts that you are offering. In the event that a relationship is not for your greater good, it may drift out of your life.

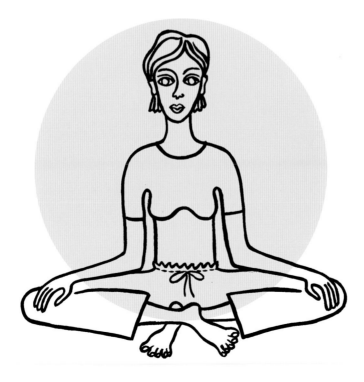

# 4 empower yourself

We involve ourselves in toxic relationships because of our own subconscious urges and engrained habits. Identifying and eliminating them will help you make rapid progress.

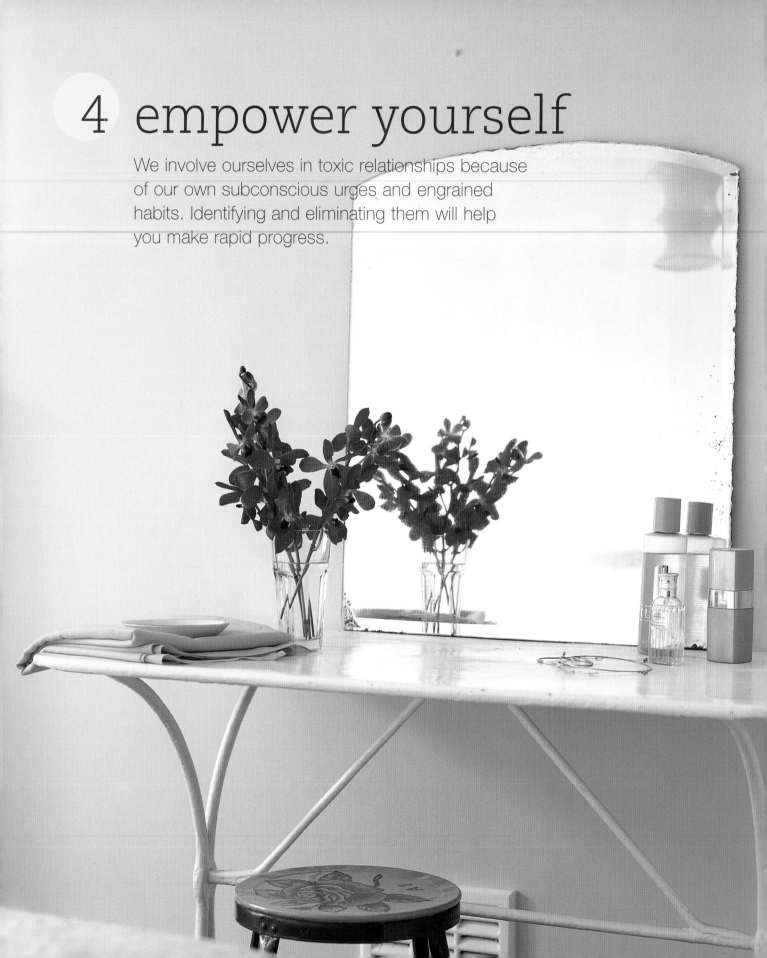

### detoxing your bad habits

Not all your relationships are with other people; you also have a relationship with yourself—and liking yourself is essential to building up self-esteem. No one knows you better than you know yourself, so, if there is something you are doing or thinking that decreases your self-respect, either stop doing it or transform it into something more acceptable.

Having a role model is a good way to stay focused on your goals. Who can you think of with qualities you would like to make your own? If you are a visual person, looking at pictures or watching videos of a role model is a positive way to keep your action plan on track. If you are especially influenced by what you hear, you may find that listening to a role model speak is more effective.

You can use the same technique to quell self-doubt or nervousness—before a job interview, for example. If you feel nervous, bring to mind someone who you think would handle the situation well—it could be someone you know personally or someone famous. Then imagine how the person would act and emulate that behavior.

### your strengths and weaknesses

Knowing your strengths and weaknesses helps you make the most of your natural talents and abilities and avoid situations that put you under unnecessary stress.

Take a sheet of paper and draw a line down the middle of it. At the top of one side write Strengths and at the top of the other Weaknesses. Then write down everything you can think of that applies to you in each of the two columns. When it comes to weaknesses, put a

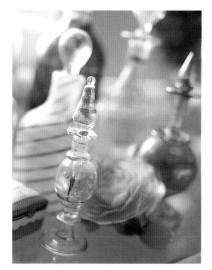

star next to any weakness that you think you can do something to improve. Then put another star against any weaknesses that you would like actively to improve in the year ahead. This exercise will give you something to work toward—and the simple fact that you have chosen to improve some areas of your life will boost your self-esteem.

### being assertive

Being assertive will not only boost your self-esteem, but will also help you transform or end relationships that are not working. Assertiveness is the art of communicating clearly and directly, without resorting to emotional manipulation or compliance. It should not be confused with aggression, which is communication without consideration for the other person's point of view.

Being assertive is about speaking up for yourself confidently and calmly when you need to let others know where you stand. For some people, being assertive is easy, but if you find it hard to get the balance right, keep practicing because the rewards are worth it.

### getting the best out of yourself

There is no point in expending a great deal of effort to detox your relationships if you are going to fall back into the same old patterns and attract more toxic people into your life.

The next page describes a number of positive habits that, if adopted, would help you get the best out of yourself and make you less likely to fall prey to other toxic relationships.

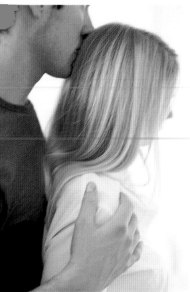

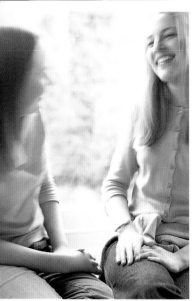

### positive habits to adopt

• Know where you are going: when you have a clear sense of who you are and have devised a well-considered goal plan, you become more difficult for other people to manipulate.

• Believe in yourself: self-belief is the first step to success. It motivates you, gives you confidence, and allows you to follow your path.

• Take responsibility: taking responsibility for your life and your actions is empowering. If you give the responsibility to someone else, you become a victim without the power to change.

• Accept your mistakes: everyone makes mistakes, but it is no use holding them against yourself. When you have done something wrong, accept it. If you can, do something about it. If you can't do something about it, forgive yourself and let it go. Remember that you learn by your mistakes and sometimes it is your mistakes that propel you further along your path of success.

• Stop putting yourself under unnecessary pressure: nobody's perfect, and it is fine to admit your faults. Even people who appear to have everything going for them have difficult times and problems of their own. Your idiosyncrasies make you unique, so don't put yourself under pressure to live up to someone else's expectations or allow anyone close to you to make you feel second best.

• Be resilient: everyone is affected sometimes by disillusionment and disappointment, and being resilient is essential if you want to keep working toward your goals. If you feel crushed by an experience, give yourself time to accept it and recover.

• Keep your sense of humor: having fun is good for you. Keeping your sense of humor can help relieve stress and lift your mood.

## boosting your
# self-respect

To win the respect of others, you must first respect yourself. Here are five tips to giving yourself a boost:

• establish boundaries—boundaries protect your energy, space, and time, and give others guidelines for how they should treat you

• surround yourself with supportive people—people who appreciate and support you will bring out the best in you

• be assertive—don't always agree to do something at the first request unless you really want to do it

• rid your life of habits, people, and situations that drain you; list all the things you put up with that bring no real benefit and take action to eliminate them

• treat yourself to something special in recognition of the fact that you are worth spoiling

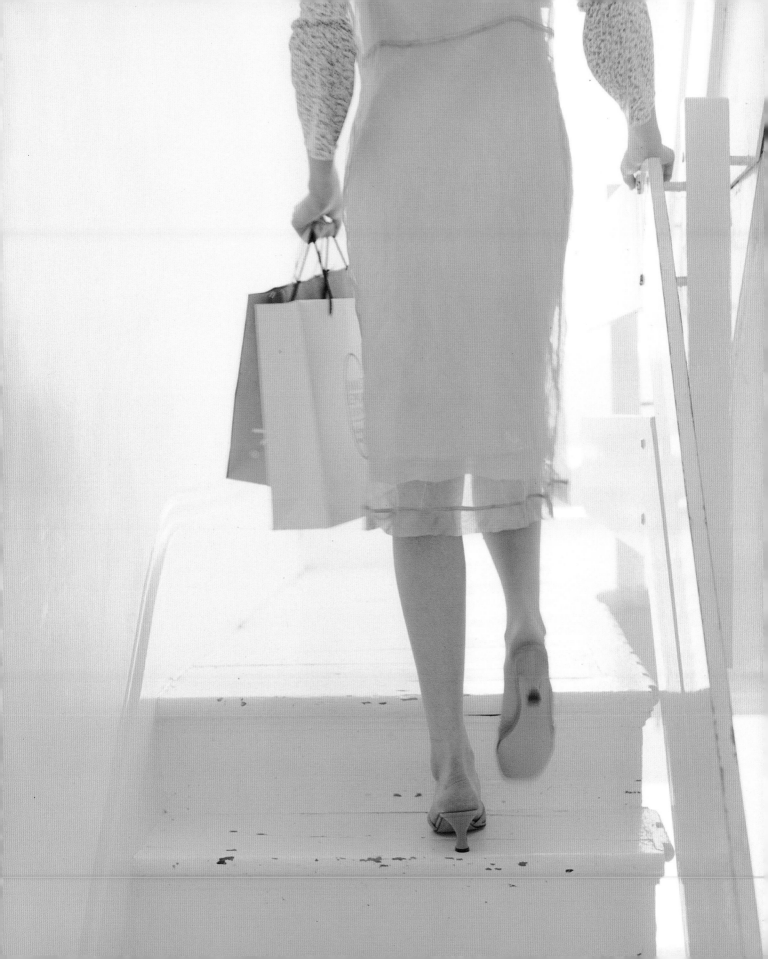

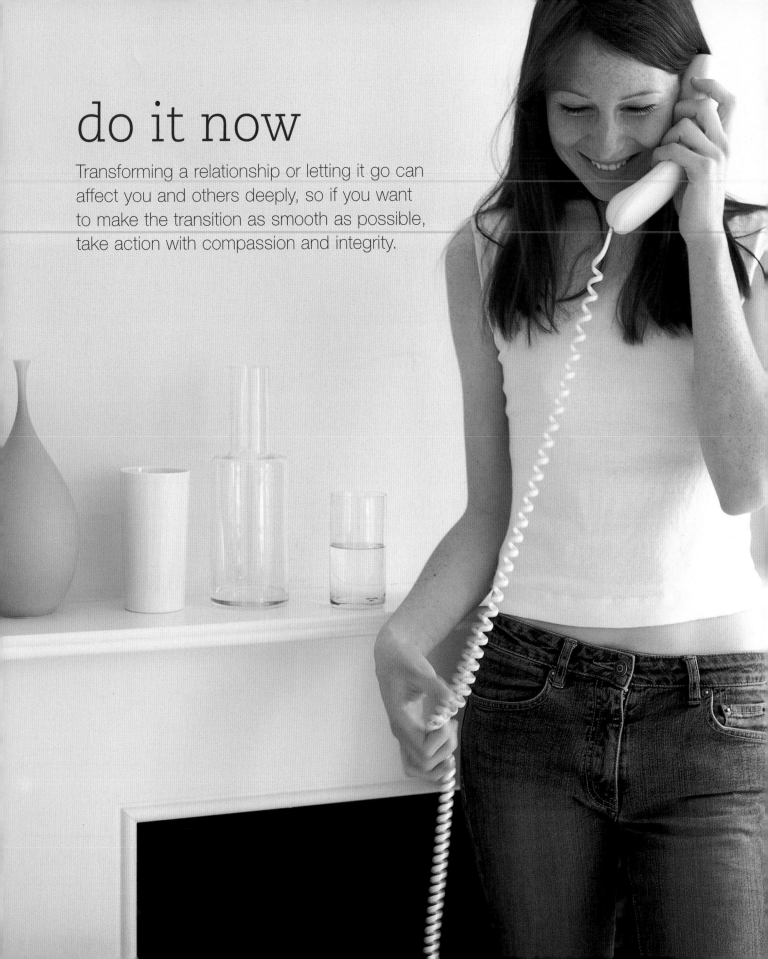

# do it now

Transforming a relationship or letting it go can affect you and others deeply, so if you want to make the transition as smooth as possible, take action with compassion and integrity.

### back to basics

The reasons why we behave as we do with certain people cannot be entirely attributed to our personality and our beliefs. Our behavior is also intricately bound up with our early relationships and our sense of love and security, so give yourself time to get to the root of the problem.

### troubleshooting

*I always feel bad about myself after an evening with Jo*
Identify what is making you feel bad and take it up with the person concerned—or, if the relationship is not worth saving, let it go.

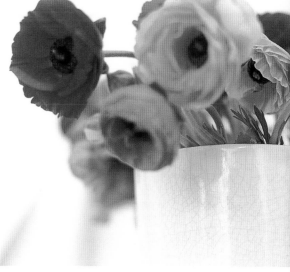

*My new boyfriend continually takes advantage of me*
Allowing others to take advantage of you reinforces low self-esteem. Decide whether you want to confront the person about this issue or let the relationship go.

*I feel envious of other people's qualities*
Identify which quality you envy in someone and learn to emulate it. Do it in a way that suits your personality, so that it doesn't look like you are copying the other person. Then, if appropriate, tell the person concerned about your admiration and explain that you would like to learn how to express the quality better.

*I always have to be careful what I say to Rose*
If you have to tailor your feelings or opinions to suit someone else, you are not free to be yourself. Decide whether the relationship is worth maintaining.

*Mike takes what he wants and gives little in return*
Mutual respect depends on achieving, over time, a balance between give and take. If you or the other person are giving or taking too much, both of you are losing out. Figure out what's upsetting the balance and decide whether you want to do something about it or let the relationship go.

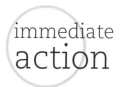

## immediate action

Pick one a relationship in your life that could be improved. It could be a relationship with your partner, a parent, a work colleague, or even a neighbor. Think about what you could do within the next 24 hours that would make a real difference. This could be saying thank you to the person concerned, inviting him or her over for coffee, writing a note, making a phone call, buying some flowers, bringing up a subject that needs discussion, or forgiving the person. Choose one task and do it now.

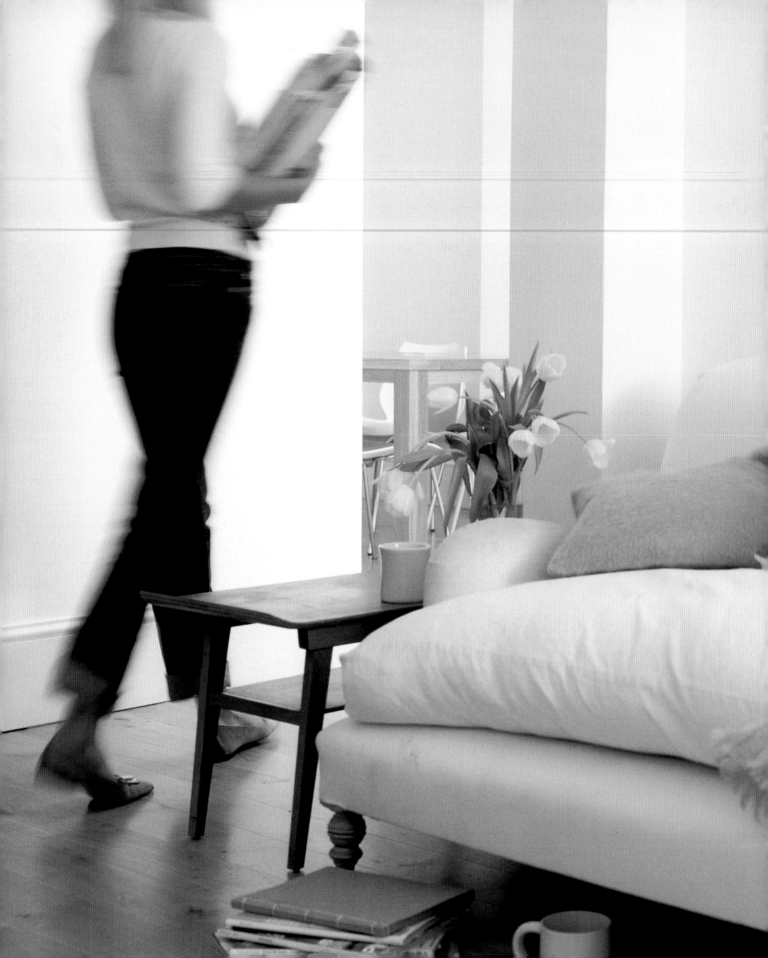

# detox
# your space

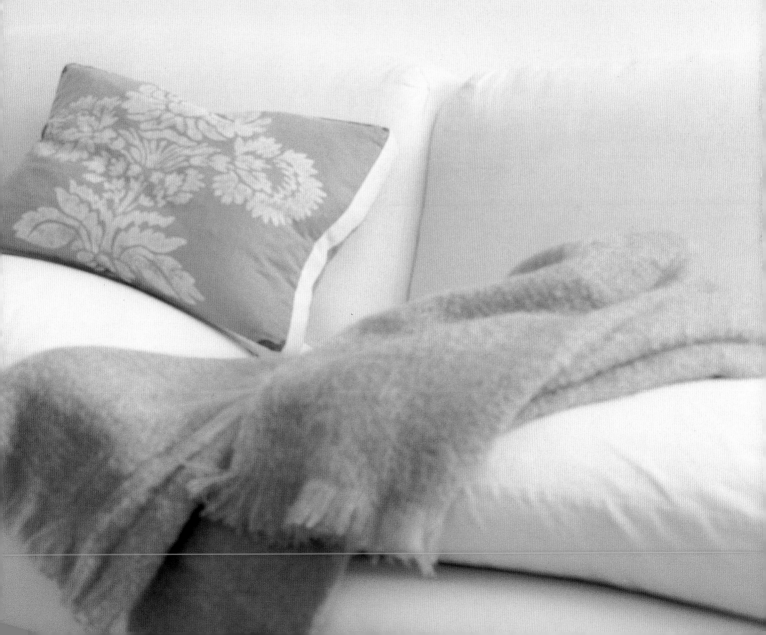

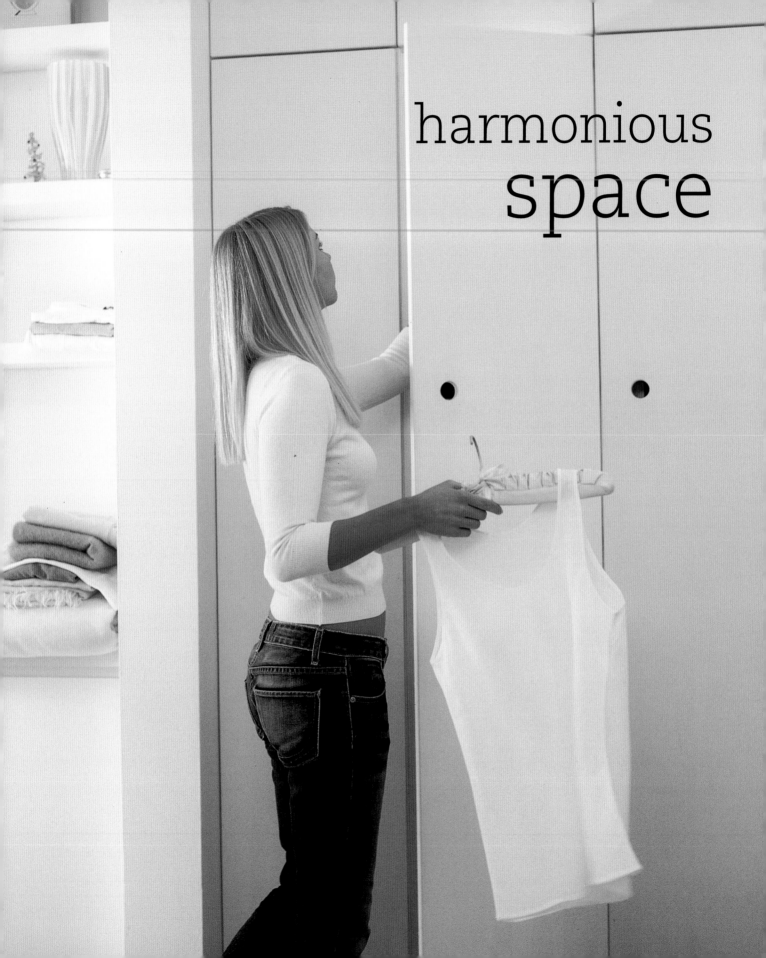

harmonious
**space**

The atmosphere of your home can affect your mental, spiritual, emotional, and physical well-being as well as your mood. A disorganized home with too much clutter consumes precious time, energy, and money. It can distract you from your real interests and damage your chances of success.

This chapter explains how to detox your space by clearing out what you don't need and becoming better organized. It describes how you can streamline your resources and reduce the amount of time and effort you put into everyday chores. It also deals with adjusting the atmosphere of your home to create an impression that makes you feel good.

If you follow the five steps in this chapter, you will begin to notice the impact your home has on yourself and others. You will learn how to banish energy that doesn't feel right to you, and how to attract positive vibrations that transform your home into an environment that is beneficial not only to you but to everyone who shares the space with you.

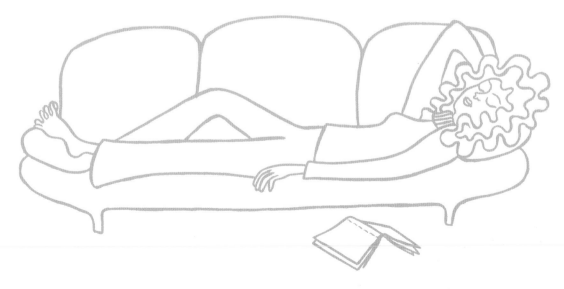

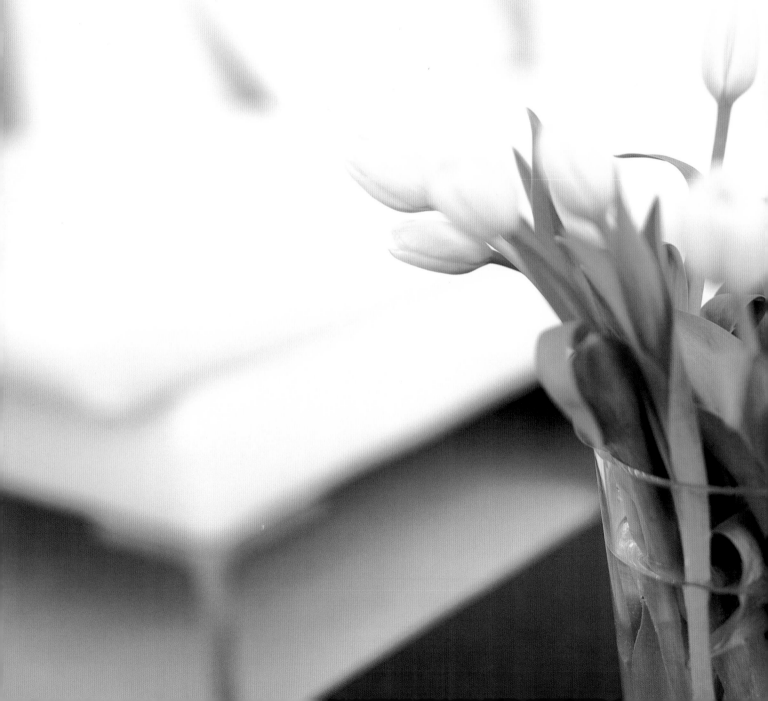

# 1 what your home says

Each person's home is a unique expression of character. Yours is no exception. Learn to read your space like a book and give prominence to the elements that give you the most pleasure and satisfaction.

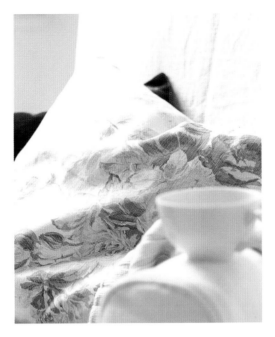

## first impressions

When people come inside your living space for the first time, they often form an immediate impression of the type of person you are from their interpretation of your surroundings. The furnishings, pictures and ornaments you choose, and how you use and combine colors, as well as the general order of the place, come together to create an overall image of who you are and what really matters to you.

It is not simply the appearance of your living space that sets the tone either. The smell, the temperature, the texture of the fabrics, and the sounds in a home all have their parts to play. These sensual elements may seem too subtle to warrant a great deal of attention—but a home that is too cold, too noisy, too uncomfortable, or which smells bad will not seem welcoming or relaxing either to you or to other people.

## establishing priorities

Understanding more about the impression your home gives will help you to decide your priorities when it comes to detoxing your living space.

For example, if your home is messy, it suggests that you are mentally rather than physically focused, and may give the impression that you are lacking in clarity and a sense of organization. On the other hand, if your home is super-tidy and well organized, it suggests that you like to be in control and dislike dwelling on emotional or psychological issues. Another strong indicator of personality is décor. Fashionable décor suggests someone who is very aware of status and image.

The person whose home has a mix of decorative styles is likely to have mixed views about life. Décor derived from a particular time period, whether it is Victorian or techno, suggests someone who believes in and lives by the values of that time.

## hidden meanings

The following survey of items that can be found in most homes and what they reveal about their owners will give you a clearer idea of the atmosphere you are creating in your own home. You can then begin to think about where you want to make changes, and consider which items you would like to keep and which you would like to let go of.

• Furniture: comfortable furniture demonstrates a desire to relax. Seating that is arranged in such a way that people can sit close together shows an enjoyment of other people's company. Furniture that has more to do with style than comfort suggests that the occupier is preoccupied with status.

• Television: a television that dominates a room relegates conversation to second place. If you put your television in a cabinet, it suggests that you like to feel a degree of control over your home and the outside world.

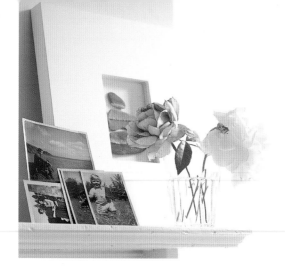

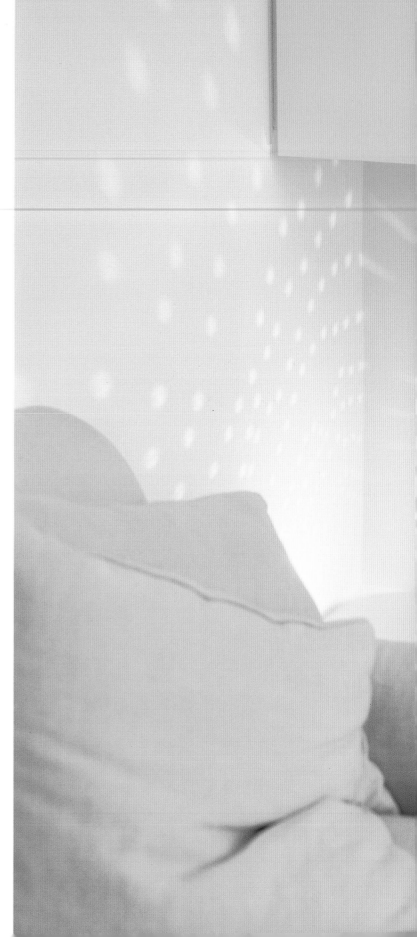

# clear out
## the past and future

Is your home full of items you no longer need from the past or things you are hoarding for the future? Both can tie you down, use up space, and impede your freedom.

If you have stacks of old letters, magazine articles, or books that you were going to read—or objects that people have given you that no longer fit into your life—it's time for a grand clear-out. The same goes for objects you have been hanging onto in case you need them and those you've kept because it would be a waste to let them go.

You don't have to get rid of everything. If you feel attached to or sentimental about something, find a place for it. If you don't want something to go to waste, give it to a thrift store, recycle it, or take it to a garage sale.

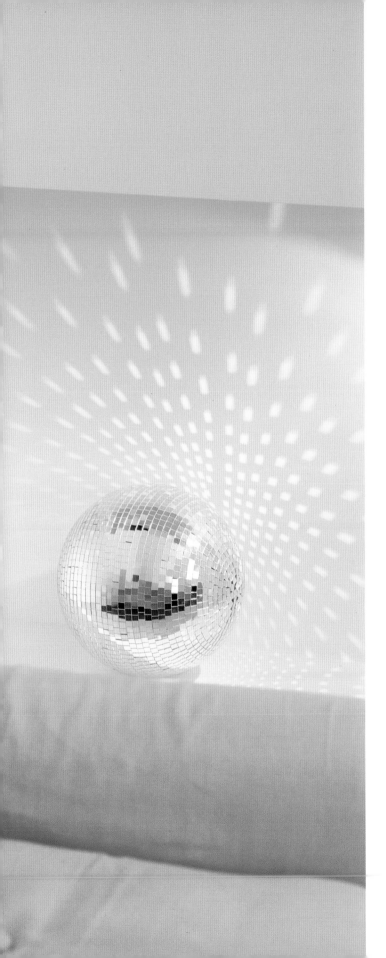

• Lighting: soft lighting indicates someone who is sensitive to the immediate environment, who may have romantic intentions, would like to feel secure, or needs to get rid of stress. People who always choose bright lights—even in the evening while they are chatting or watching television—are likely to be less sensitive to their surroundings and the people around them, and may be particularly focused on intellectual pursuits.

• Music: the style of music you prefer gives clues to your emotional life. Hard rock suggests someone who likes to portray themselves as tough and resilient. People who like pop music generally put a high value on feeling part of their peer group and the community. A preference for classical music indicates someone with deep emotions who is not easily swayed by fashion.

Choosing to play background music, particularly when others are present, is typical of people who like to set the tone of their home; they know how to manipulate their environment and often like to take charge.

• Plants: people who like to cultivate plants in the home frequently enjoy nurturing not only their environment, but also the people around them. Artificial plants show someone who may be willing to settle for second best.

• Pictures: a fondness for displaying photographs often reveals the need to be part of a family or a peer group (depending on who is shown in them). Paintings or illustrations of people may indicate that the owner enjoys the company of the type of people represented in the pictures. Pictures of children, animals, or plants show a soft spot for the type of living thing depicted. Pictures of houses or landscapes often evoke the type of atmosphere that makes the occupiers of the home feel most comfortable.

Abstract pictures indicate someone who may have mental or emotional issues to resolve. Abstracts are also favored by people who would like to make their emotional or creative presence felt, although they may not be particularly sociable.

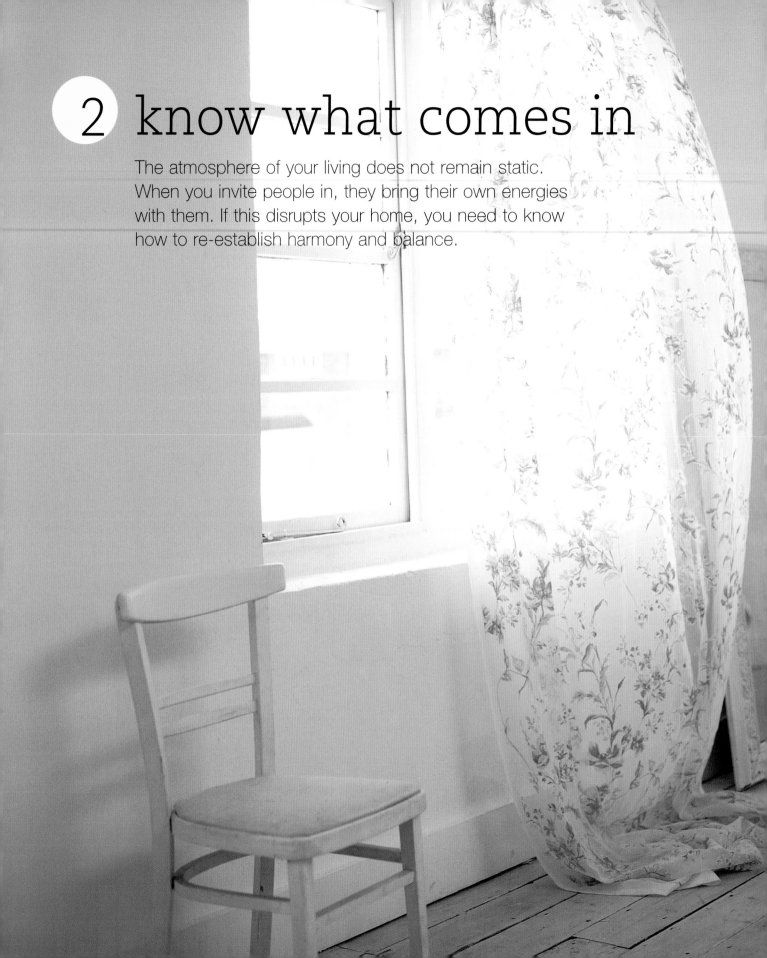

# 2 know what comes in

The atmosphere of your living does not remain static.
When you invite people in, they bring their own energies
with them. If this disrupts your home, you need to know
how to re-establish harmony and balance.

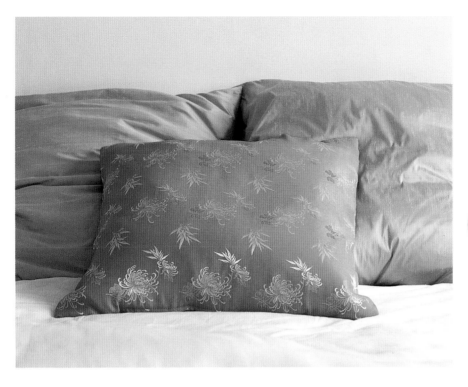

# the mood

To bring an immediate change of mood, follow these steps:

• create some sort of order; if you have too much clutter to clear up immediately, simply put everything that needs sorting or tidying into a few plastic bags or boxes

• clean the kitchen floor, make the bed, or plump up the cushions

• open the windows to let in fresh air, change the temperature, and generally move the energy around

• add a few drops of essential oil to an aromatherapy burner or to water in an atomizer that can be sprayed around the home

• put on some soothing music

### restoring peace and optimism

The intensely personal nature of your home means that you should be aware of who and what comes into it.

When you invite people into your personal living space for the first time, you are making yourself vulnerable by letting them know more about you. More importantly, the people who come into your space bring with them their own personal energy, which can sometimes change the atmosphere dramatically.

There are some people who have a knack of creating a feeling of stress or uneasiness for those around them, and when this happens in your home, it disturbs the feeling of harmony, peace, and optimism. Sometimes a bad atmosphere is created by the people who live in a home and lingers after an argument or when something unhappy has occurred.

You will know if the energy of your home needs attention if you feel uncomfortable and unsettled when you look around. In such circumstances, a quick detox can help you to feel more in control of the situation and in a better position to cope (see above right).

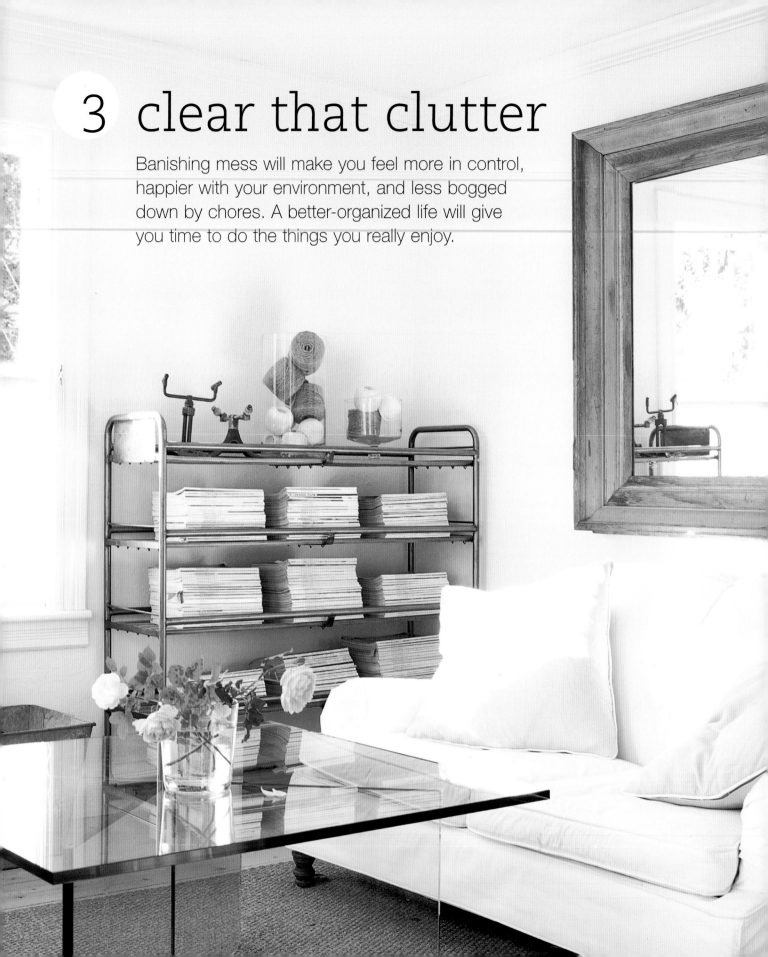

# 3 clear that clutter

Banishing mess will make you feel more in control, happier with your environment, and less bogged down by chores. A better-organized life will give you time to do the things you really enjoy.

### the clutter mountain

Do you have magazines that need to be read, letters that should be answered, drawers and closets that could be better organized—or just too much stuff hanging around? If so, clutter is part of your life, and you need to deal with it. Ignoring clutter leads to procrastination, loss of control, money wasting, and increased stress levels.

### a methodical approach

Start by identifying the areas in your house that need work. On a legal pad, write down a heading for each section of your home, then walk around your house and mark all the areas that need to be cleared out and detoxed. This could be an entire room or a particular area, such as a closet or drawer.

Instead of trying to detox the entire space at once—and running out of time and energy—start small. Once you have listed the clutter areas, you can make a detox plan by allocating enough time to tackle each section of your home and marking it on your calendar. As you complete and check off each section, you should feel good about yourself—and this should help strengthen your resolve and stop you from feeling defeated.

The next stage is to find seven large bags or boxes and a garbage sack, mark them as shown on right, and sort your clutter into the respective containers. Then write on the box or bag a deadline by which you intend to have the items in the box or bag sorted out, and also how much time you have allocated to do this sorting. Put these dates on your calendar, too.

If you regularly have a lot of clutter to deal with, you could create a permanent place to keep pending clutter. But to stop the contents of this box or bag from building up, schedule a regular time to go through it—perhaps half an hour a week or an evening once a month.

### keeping on top of clutter

For most people, clutter is part of everyday life, so if you want to stay on top of it and keep your space detoxed, you should be aware of where the clutter in your life comes from, what control you have over it, and the ways you can keep it under control.

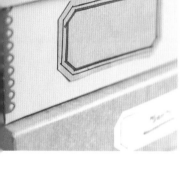

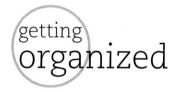

the clutter took time to build up and it will take time to clear

## getting organized

Mark and fill your bags and boxes as follows:

- **put away:** any items that have a place and need to be put away

- **create a place:** items that you want to keep but have no place for

- **action:** articles to read, letters that need answering, and so on

- **repair:** anything that needs to be altered, repaired, or cleaned

- **pass on:** items to donate to a charity or secondhand shop

- **recycle**

- **not sure:** any items that you cannot decide about

- **trash**

### know the reasons for your clutter

If you are burdened by a large amount of clutter, ask yourself these questions to find out why:

*Am I too impulsive about bringing items into my home?*

*Am I buying items to make me feel better about myself?*

*Do I hang onto things for too long?*

*Am I hanging onto things because I have inherited or been given them, even though I don't really like them?*

*Do I keep a lot of things in case they might be useful in the future?*

*Do I buy or keep things to maintain my status or because they are fashionable?*

### a control strategy

If you have a clutter problem, always ask yourself three questions before bringing a new item into your home. Will this make a positive difference to my life? Have I got room for it? Am I prepared to let go of something to make room for it? All items that have already found their way into your home should have a place to live. If they haven't, get hold of some easily accessible storage such as accordion files, drawers, and boxes, and put the things away. There should also be places for in-between items—clothes that you have worn and plan to wear again soon or magazines that are half read, for instance. If everything has somewhere to go, there is no excuse for having it hanging around.

Get into the habit of putting things away as soon as you have finished with them—for example, when your clean washing is dry, put it in the drawers or closet immediately. When you have finished looking at a book, put it back on the shelf. When someone gives you their telephone number, write it in your address book.

Allocate yourself regular "mail and paperwork time": this is essential if you want to keep on top of your correspondence and make sure your paperwork is well organized and filed.

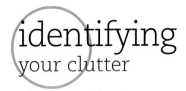

# identifying
## your clutter

To determine whether something counts as clutter, look at the item and ask yourself these questions:

• does this feel like me?

• does this make me feel good?

• can I genuinely see myself using it again?

• if I let it go and then need it or something similar later, will it be easy to find a replacement?

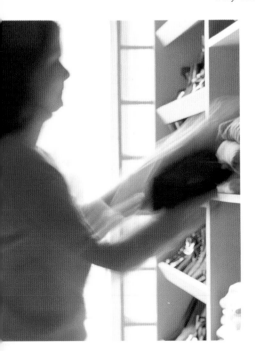

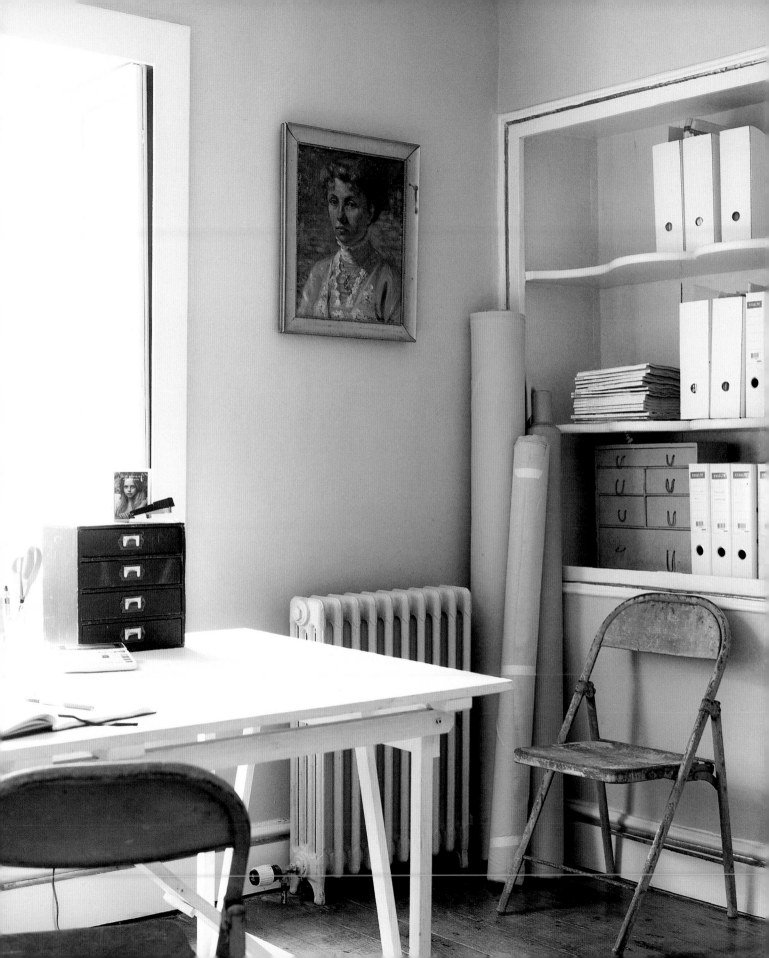

# 4 create an energy flow

You may sense that the atmosphere in your home is in some way stressful or stagnant. If you do have this experience, the time has come to generate a positive flow of energy.

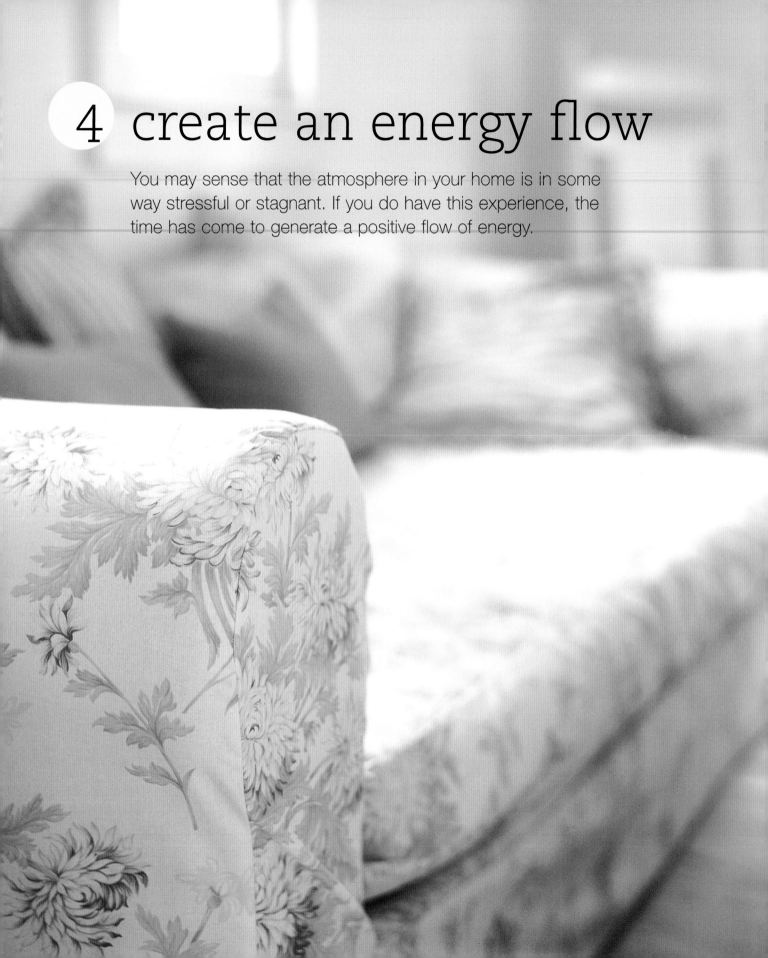

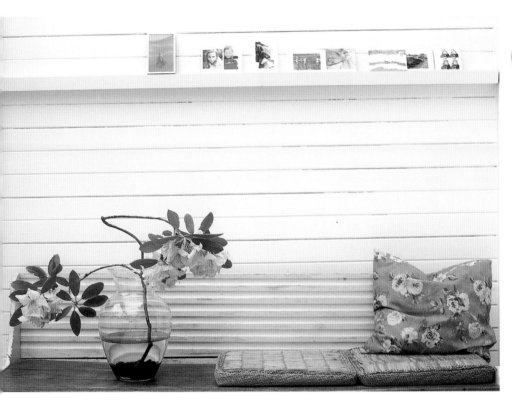

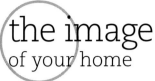

# the image
of your home

To refine your awareness of the impression your home gives, ask yourself the following questions:

• how organized is my home?

• how does it smell?

• how does it feel?

• do I like the color scheme?

• do I like the furniture?

• do I like the pictures?

• do I like the lighting?

## reaping the benefits

Once you have started to rid your home of clutter, you should begin to experience the benefits of the detoxing process. The atmosphere should feel lighter and less stressed. You may find that you have more time on your hands—or perhaps you feel more confident because you have become better organized.

Every home has its own character, and thinking of your home as space that represents you makes it easier to decide how you could improve the atmosphere. Your home is the place you go to recharge your batteries, to relax, and to be private, and it should enable you to do these things with ease. It should also be somewhere where you can let your intuition, inspiration, and creativity flow. Above all, it should be somewhere you like to be.

## how you want to be seen

Before you make any changes, you should be aware of the image you would like your home to portray. Start by considering what impression a stranger would have upon entering your home. Think about how you feel when you enter each room. Is the atmosphere relaxed, tense, happy, or something else?

The next step is to decide what sort of image you would ideally like to convey. This might be calm and relaxed, comfortable and practical, sophisticated and sexy, unusual and interesting—or perhaps a mixture of different qualities.

A harmonious home is a place that represents its occupants faithfully—so, if you are not sure about the image you should be aiming to create, consider the people who live in your home, write down two words that describe positive qualities associated with each of them, and give some thought to these qualities.

If you find that the people you live with have very different tastes and interests, give them specific areas in which to express themselves. For example, children could choose designs for their own bedrooms, or you and your partner could agree on a bookshelf or wall to devote to a specific interest.

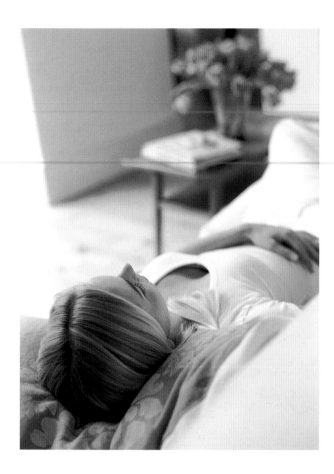

to detox your
bedroom and
keep it clear,
give priority
to storage

## making the right impression

For your home to have a positive atmosphere, it needs to function well. When deciding what changes to make, consider the following points.

• The front door: your front door separates you from the outside world. When someone comes to visit you, it is the first part of your home they look at. The color and style of your door should represent the occupants.

• The entrance hall: it is worth putting effort into the appearance of your entrance hall since it gives visitors the first real indication of the sort of person you are. This is usually an area that sees a lot of human traffic, so try to keep it clear.

• The living room: the living room is the most public part of your home and often the most revealing. The atmosphere in the room will affect how relaxed you are and how you relate to your visitors and the other occupants of your home.

• The dining room: eating together is one of the few daily rituals still practiced by many families. To get the most out of your dining area, the chairs should be comfortable so the diners can take their time to eat, digest their meal well, and communicate with each other.

• The bedroom: as the last place you see at night, a bedroom needs to be relaxing and convey a sense of order. It is also the first place you see in the morning, so it should be uplifting, too.

• The study or office: a clear desk will help you to keep a clear mind while you are working, encouraging productivity, creativity, and good organization.

• The kitchen: the kitchen is one of the most functional areas of your home and is closely associated on both a conscious and subconscious level with wellbeing. It should be well organized and clean, with good lighting.

• The bathroom: as the room where you spend time getting ready to face the world and winding down (particularly if you have a bath), a bathroom should be functional, soothing, and refreshing.

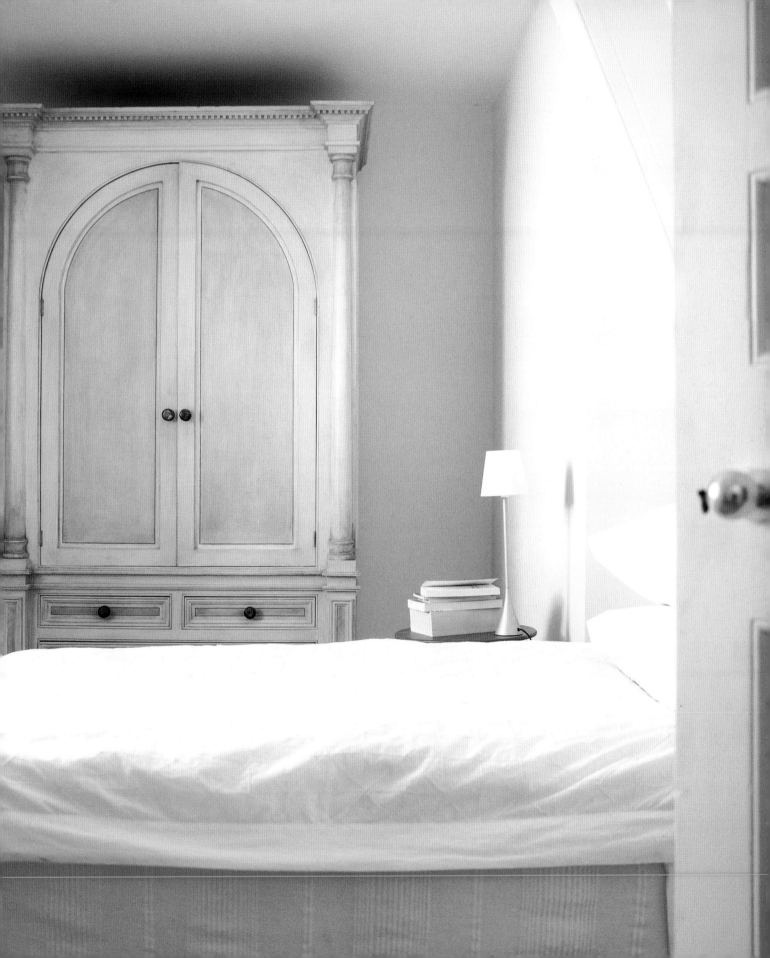

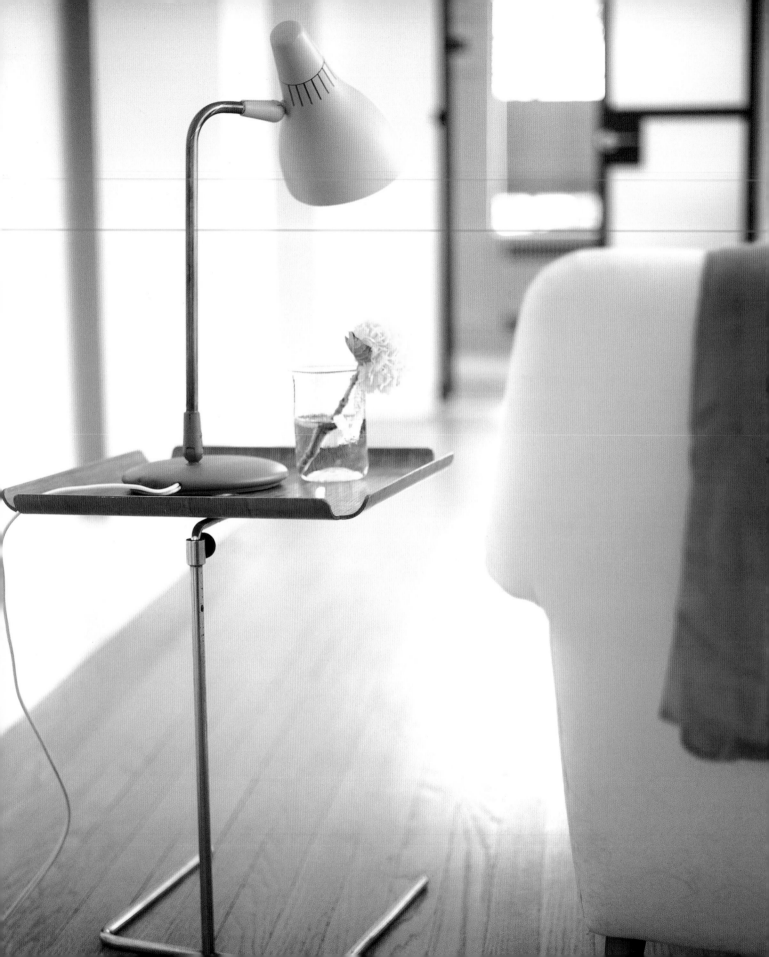

subtle use of
light, color,
and mirrors
gives a breath
of fresh air

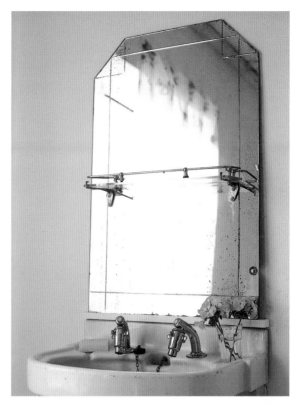

## five quick fixes

There are a number of things you can do to make an instant difference to your home without investing too much time and money.

• Lighting: use lamps to introduce an atmosphere of relaxation and intimacy. Candles are particularly good for creating a relaxing and romantic atmosphere.

• Mirrors: mirrors can be used to double the size of a room and create a sense of light, openness, and space. They are particularly effective if you feel oppressed by your environment.

• Pictures: you can set the scene for a particular room by choosing pictures or photographs that represent the image you are trying to portray. For example, if you want to create a peaceful environment, you might choose a picture of green pastures or wild flowers.

• Plants: plants are aesthetically pleasing and show that you care for your environment. They can also swiftly improve the quality of air in your home.

• Colors: the two or three main colors you choose in any room of your home to cover the largest areas will set the tone for that room. Warm colors are associated with an intimate environment, while cool colors create an impression of distance.

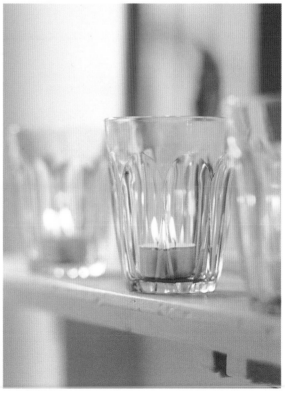

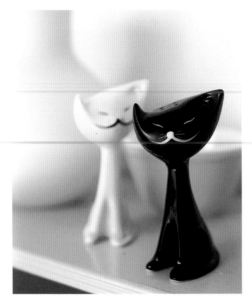

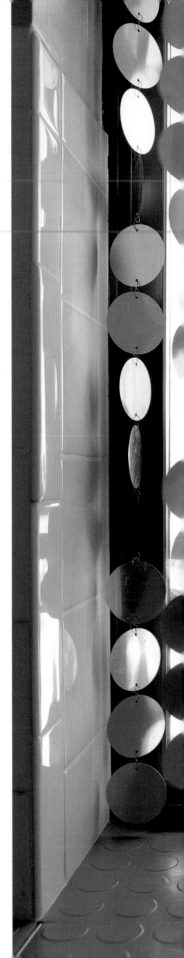

### the language of symbolism

Animals, plants, and the natural elements have been used symbolically for centuries in many different cultures to attract certain qualities into people's lives. These symbols not only have a mystical power that has become established over time, but they can also be put to more practical use. When you place a symbolic object or plant somewhere obvious in your house, whenever you see it you are reminded of the quality it represents. Being conscious of that quality helps you to integrate it into your life.

# animals
## as symbols

Some animal figures or pictures attract certain qualities:

• a cat attracts sensuality, pride, and comfort

• a dog attracts loyalty, reliability, and protection

• a fox attracts cunning, agility, and self-reliance

• a horse attracts persuasiveness, popularity, and accomplishment

• a lion attracts bravery and nobility

• a pig attracts luxury, indulgence, and inquisitiveness

• a rooster attracts resilience, pioneering, and confidence

• a snake attracts sexuality, mystery, and psychic ability

• a tortoise attracts relaxation, endurance, and thoughtfulness

### the natural world

If you would like to attract a particular quality or feeling into your home, consider picking an ornament or picture that represents one of the following elements.

• Wood: growth, learning, and productivity. Ornaments that represent wood are plants, wooden objects, pictures of trees or landscapes, and the color green.

• Fire: warmth, passion, and energy. Ornaments that represent fire are candles, lamps, symbols of the sun, pictures of fire, and the color red.

• Earth: nurturing, support, and practicality. Ornaments representing the earth are terracotta and pottery, stones, square shapes, and the colors orange and brown.

• Air: spirit, mind, and freedom. Ornaments representing air include fans, angels, items such as mobiles that hang from the ceiling, and the colors white and blue.

• Metal: creativity, strength and action. Ornaments that represent metal are metal objects, coins, clocks, and the colors silver and gray.

• Water: understanding, purity, and tranquility. Ornaments that represent water are mirrors, glass, fish tanks, pictures of water, and the colors blue and green.

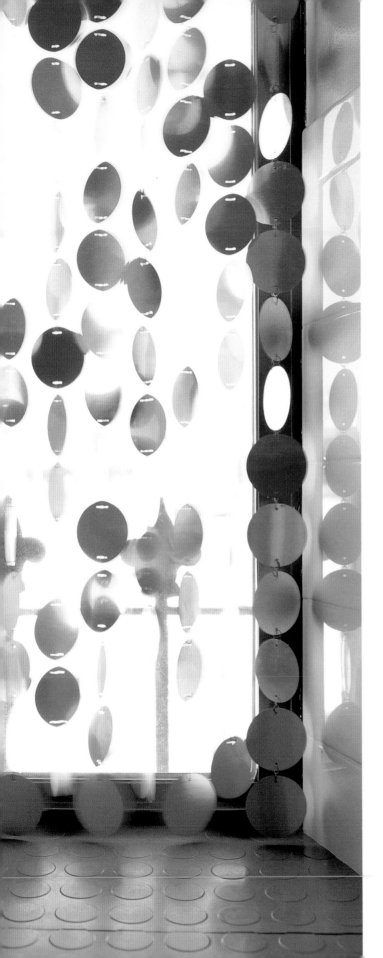

# plants
## as symbols

Plants have also been used for centuries to represent and attract certain qualities:

• a peace lily brings peace

• aloe vera is associated with healing

• a money plant attracts wealth and long life

• a spider plant brings choices and resilience

• cactus wards off negativity—but don't have a cactus in the bedroom or it may repel other people

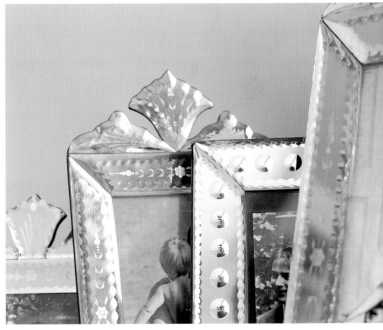

# 5 cleanse and refresh

You may have cleared your clutter, moved your furniture around, and changed the color of your walls—and yet the atmosphere in your home still doesn't feel right. If this is the case, you need to cleanse and refresh the energy in your home.

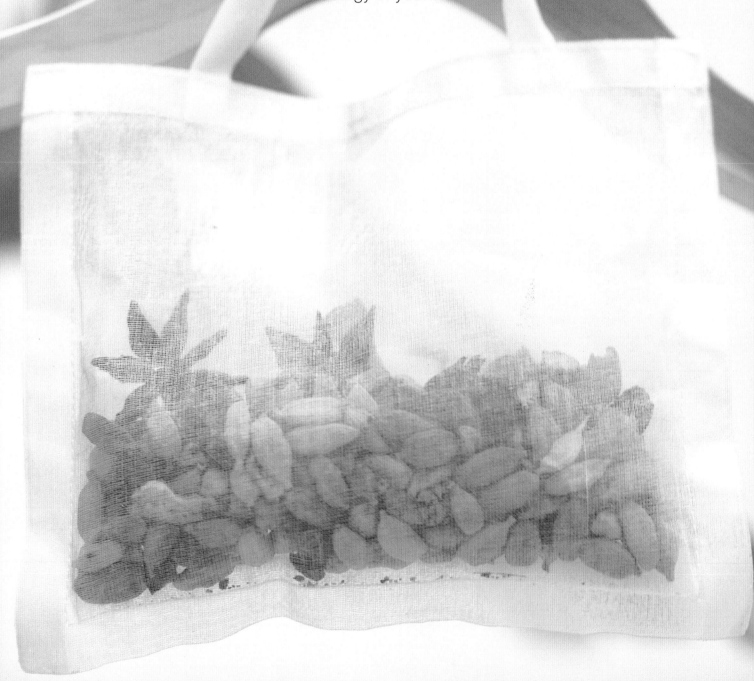

# protect your home

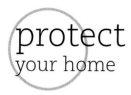

Simple ways to protect the energy in your home from bad influences include using symbols of animals and plants (see pages 116–117).

For example, placing two animal figures such as lions, dragons, or dogs either side of the entrance to your garden or your front door is a traditional way to protect your property.

Alternatively, you could plant a rowan tree or a holly bush in your yard. Both species are said to have protective energies.

### claiming your territory

There are many traditional ways to clear the energy in your home. They are particularly useful if your home needs revitalizing, or if you move into a new house and want to detox the old atmosphere and claim your new territory as your own.

### creating a new sanctuary

After making sure that your clutter has been cleared (see pages 106–109), you can thoroughly purge and refresh your home to establish a sanctuary. Do this by following the steps outlined below. When you have finished, let the atmosphere settle. It won't be until you resume your day-to-day life that your home will start to feel truly familiar again.

• Open a window in every room. This will encourage the air to circulate and allow any stale air to disperse.

• Carry out a thorough spring clean of all the surfaces, fabrics, windows, mirrors, and anything else that could do with cleaning.

• Change the smell of each room or each floor by burning some incense. Alternatively, you could use an aromatherapy burner or an atomizer filled with water and a few drops of essential oil. Sage oil or citrus oils are particularly effective for cleansing the atmosphere (see pages 64–65 for more details). You may also decide to do some cooking in the kitchen to change the smell. Garlic and onion are traditional cleansers—both for the body and for the atmosphere. You could also make some real coffee; the smell will lift the atmosphere.

• Place fresh flowers or plants around the house.

• Change the feeling of the house by playing uplifting or soothing music.

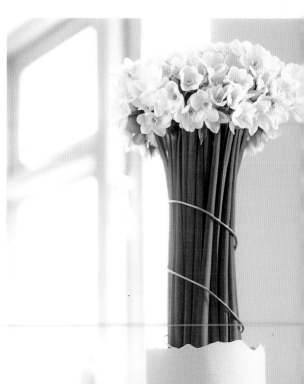

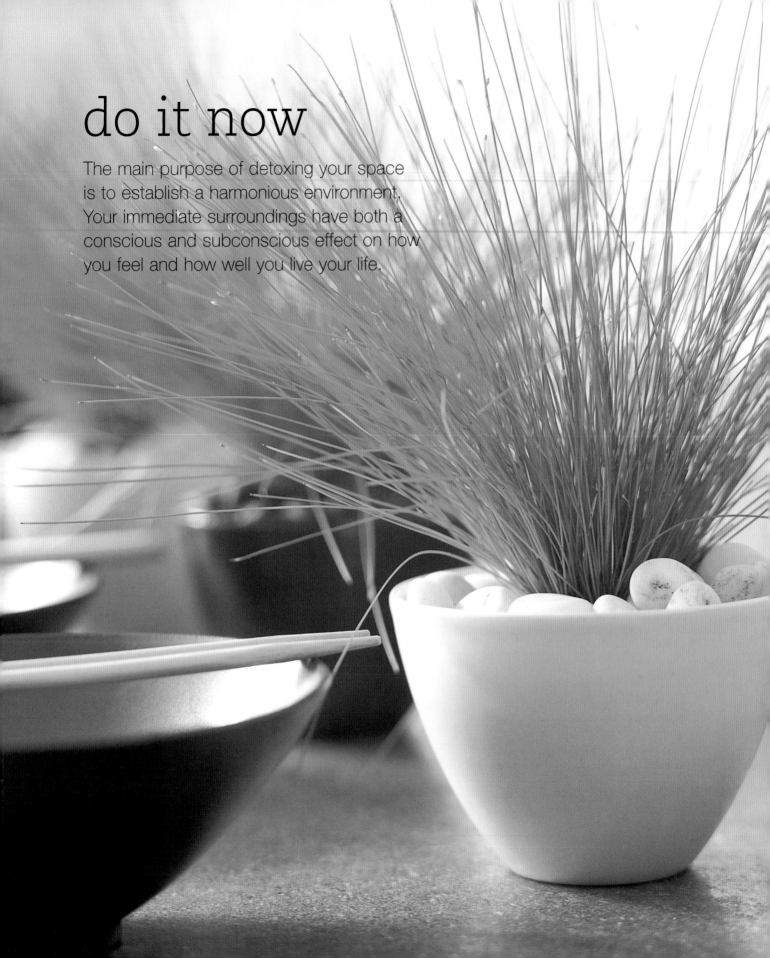

# do it now

The main purpose of detoxing your space is to establish a harmonious environment. Your immediate surroundings have both a conscious and subconscious effect on how you feel and how well you live your life.

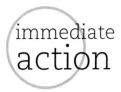

# immediate action

Pick an area of your home that's in need of improvement. It could be your bedroom, the hall or a corner of the kitchen or bathroom. Think about what you could do within the next 24 hours that would make a positive difference to that area. This could be anything from clearing clutter, rearranging your possessions, or cleaning the windows to introducing a symbolic picture or plant. Choose one or more tasks that would have an instantaneous effect on this part of your home and do it now.

## a new freedom

If you are the type of person who collects possessions almost without trying, clearing your clutter could take time. You may have to have more than one attempt at it before you are satisfied with the results. But once you have finished the task, you should feel a new freedom. Remember that it is not only the function of your home that's important, but also how your home feels to you.

## troubleshooting

*I am overwhelmed by clutter*
Break the clutter in your home into small manageable types, then pick a type to work on that, once cleared, will make the most obvious difference to your life.

*The prospect of clearing up bores me*
Decide how much time you are willing to spend clearing up, then choose something enjoyable to listen to while you sort out the mess.

*I feel guilty about getting rid of gifts*
Gifts that you don't like or that are of no use to you would be better off being given to someone who would appreciate them. If you really don't want to let a gift go, make sure that it has a place to live in your home.

*How can I change the image of my home without spending too much?*
Applying a fresh coat of paint, adding a few plants, or covering your sofa or bed with an attractive sheet of fabric are among the quickest and cheapest ways to change the image of your home.

*I feel that the atmosphere in my home needs a very powerful detox*
A traditional cleansing method is to sprinkle a handful of salt (sea salt is good if you can get it) at the front and back entrances to purify and keep away any negative energies. Leave it there overnight and sweep it up in the morning.

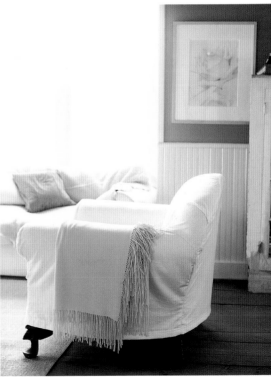

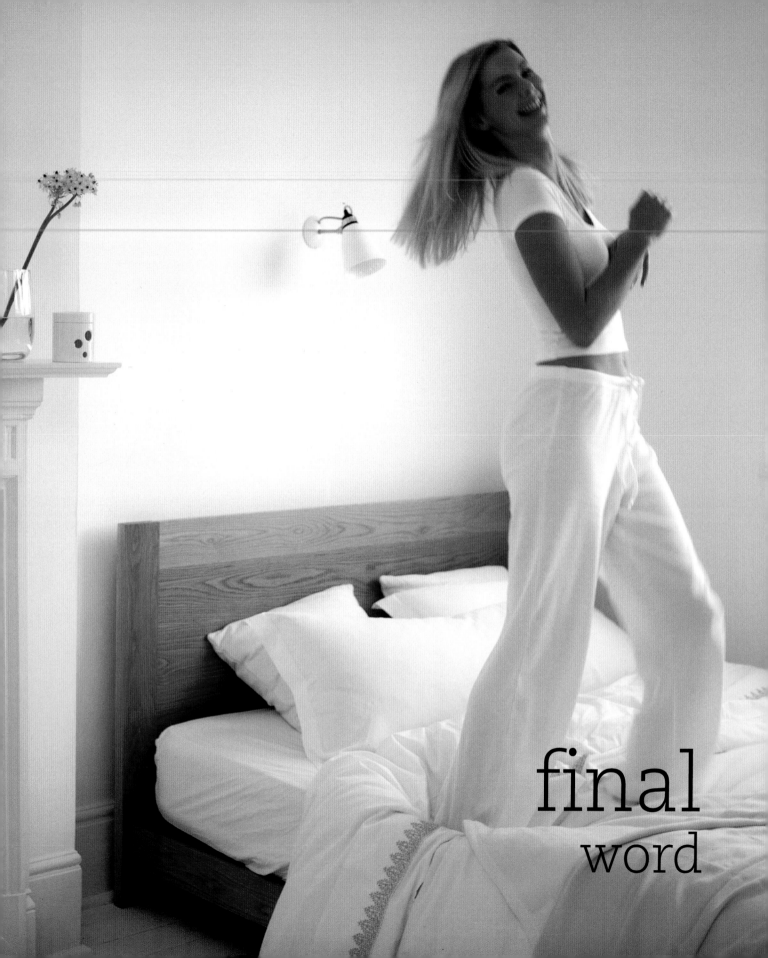

final
word

Making changes to your life takes time and patience. You may be dealing with habits and routines that have built up over a long period, sometimes many years. Commitment and persistence are essential to getting the results you want, but it's normal to fall back into your old ways now and again, so go easy on yourself.

One way to stay on top of your detox program is to devise a list of realistic daily goals. Even if you achieve just one goal on your list each day, you will be making some progress. If you have trouble accomplishing your goals during the day even though they seem realistic, it may be useful to analyze where your time is going.

If you do the exercise described on page 124 for three to seven days, it will give you a clearer understanding of how effectively you use your time. It will also help you to think of ways to free up more time for yourself, perhaps through delegation or better organization.

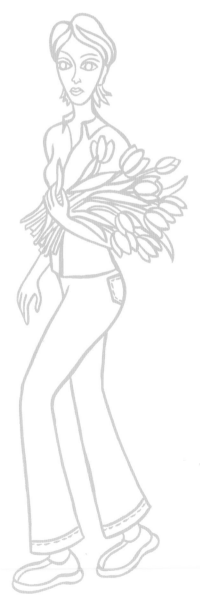

### where is your time going?

Take a large piece of paper and draw a line down the middle of it. At the top of the left-hand column, write the heading "My goals for today" and down the left-hand side of this column make a list of the hours of the day. Start with the hour nearest to the time you get up—7 A.M., for example—and below that write 8 A.M., 9 A.M., and so on, until you have written down all the hours up to the time you go to sleep. At the head of the right-hand column, write "What I did today."

At the beginning of your day (or the night before), write down the goals you would like to achieve during that day and plot them in the left-hand column next to the time you think you might be able to accomplish them by. As the day progresses, fill in what you are doing with your time in the right-hand column.

When you have done this exercise for at least three days, you should be able to identify areas where you waste time or could improve your efficiency. It could be that you are simply trying to fit too much into your day—in which case perhaps you should cut back on your activities and simplify your schedule.

If you are genuinely short of time, but still want to accomplish a number of goals, maybe you can organize your time to complete two goals at once. For example, if you need some exercise and also want to spend more time with your partner or family, you could consider doing something sporty with them, maybe a bike ride or a swim. Maybe you want to expand your social circle and also want to learn a new skill. In this case, an evening class could help you to achieve both goals at once. With a little thought, you could double your efficiency.

### make your detox happy and rewarding

Don't underestimate the importance of happiness. Being happy can keep you young, release stress, and attract positive experiences. One of the most common reasons why people revert to their old habits and routines is that they start to feel discouraged and disheartened.

Following a detox and goal plan can take hard work, commitment, and persistence, and you are much more likely to stick to your plan if you feel positive about it—so find a way of making your detox enjoyable and reward yourself when you have completed important tasks.

### have a support network

There is nothing like someone else's critism or negativity to put a dampener on your plans. If your detox and goal plan involves giving up or cutting down on an addiction

success is far more likely if you feel good about what you're doing

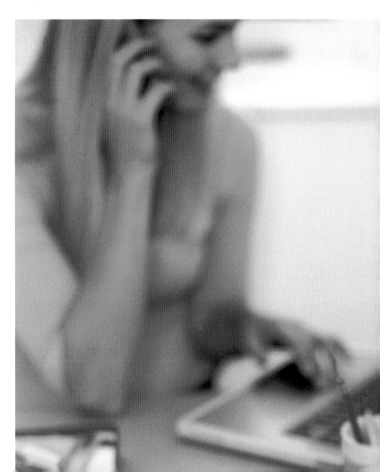

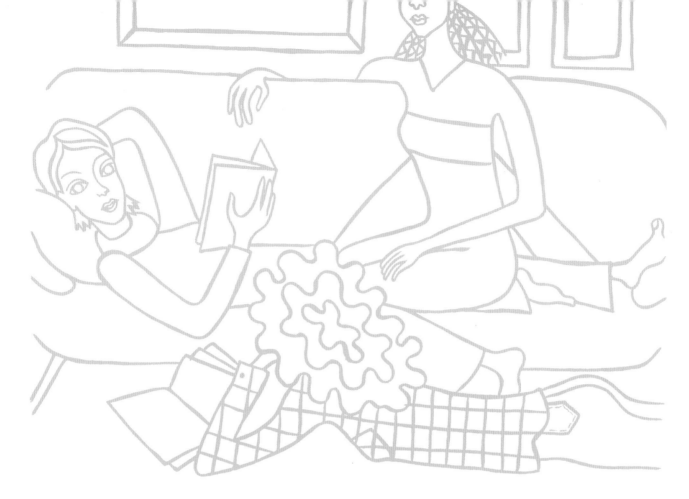

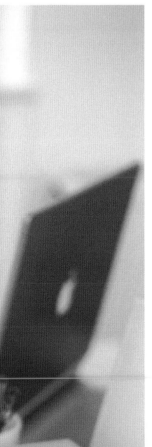

such as smoking, drinking, or shopping, or involves letting go of or transforming a close relationship, it is advisable to seek professional help or to join a support group. Sometimes it helps to find someone who has similar goals to you, so that you can cheer each other on. Get the support of family, friends, and colleagues if you can—but don't share your plan with someone who you suspect does not have your best interests at heart.

## what if you do nothing?

Finally, it is worth considering what there is to lose if you choose not to detox your life and follow your goal plan. Although you may be reasonably satisfied with your life as it is, you could miss out on opportunities and experiences, and fail to accomplish things you would like to do because you are not on top of your life.

Remember that taking or not taking action always has consequences. This is your life, and only you can decide what is important and appropriate for you.

*So—good luck!*

# one step
## at a time

Many of us suffer from an all-or-nothing mentality, which means that we either want to detox our life thoroughly and immediately, or we don't want to bother because the task seems overwhelming. If this applies to you, remind yourself that it can take time to transform your vision into reality. Take one small step at a time and bear in mind that each step is bringing you closer to achieving your grand plan.

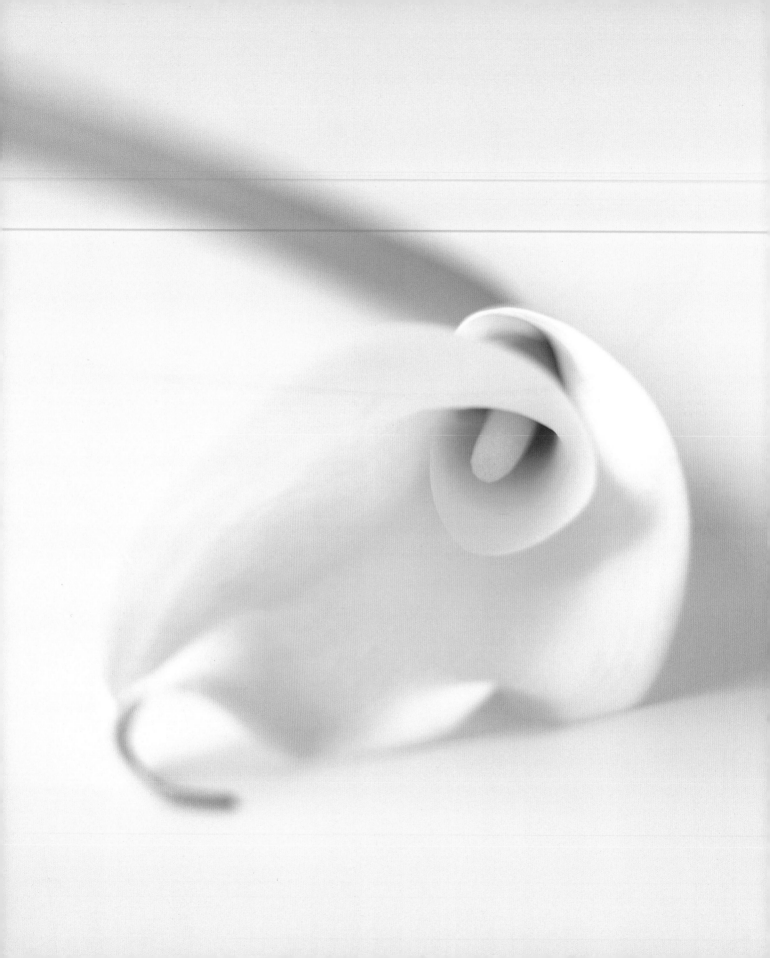

# picture credits

All photography by Polly Wreford unless otherwise specified.

Key: ph=photographer a=above, b=below, r=right, l=left, c=center.

Endpapers ph Tom Leighton; 1 ph David Montgomery; 4–5 ph Dan Duchars; 6 ph Ray Main/Robert Callender & Elizabeth Ogilvie's studio in Fife designed by John C Hope Architects; 12 Francesca Mills' house in London; 14 Clare Nash's house in London; 15b ph Dan Duchars; 18 ph Debi Treloar; 22–23 Mary Foley's house in Connecticut; 28–29 ph Andrew Wood/Guido Palau's house in North London, designed by Azman Owens Architects; 31 ph David Montgomery; 36 ph David Montgomery; 38 & 39b ph Debi Treloar; 39a ph David Montgomery; 40 Kimberley Watson's house in London; 41l ph Simon Upton; 41r ph Peter Cassidy; 42 ph David Brittain; 43 ph David Montgomery; 44–45 ph Debi Treloar; 46 ph Andrew Wood; 47–49 ph Debi Treloar; 52 ph Tom Leighton; 53l ph David Montgomery; 53c&r ph Debi Treloar; 54 & 55b ph Andrew Wood; 55a ph Christopher Drake; 56 ph Jan Baldwin; 61b ph David Montgomery; 62 ph Caroline Arber; 63l ph David Montgomery; 63c ph Chris Everard/the Sugarman–Behun house on Long Island; 63r ph Debi Treloar; 64–66 ph David Montgomery; 67 ph Henry Bourne; 70 ph Dan Duchars; 73 ph Catherine Gratwicke/Lulu Guinness's home in London; 78 ph Dan Duchars; 80c ph Sandra Lane; 80b ph David Loftus; 81 ph Tom Leighton; 84 ph Dan Duchars; 86 ph Debi Treloar; 88–89 ph Dan Duchars; 90 Clare Nash's house in London; 91 ph Chris Everard/Lulu Guinness's home in London; 92b, 93 & 94 ph Dan Duchars; 100 ph Alan Williams/Jennifer & Geoffrey Symonds' apartment in New York designed by Jennifer Post Design; 102–103 ph Andrew Wood/Guido Palau's house in North London, designed by Azman Owens Architects; 104 The Sawmills Studios; 105 Clare Nash's house in London; 106 ph Jan Baldwin/Mona Nerenberg and Lisa Bynon's house in Sag Harbor; 108 ph Andrew Wood; 109 Lena Proudlock's house in Gloucestershire; 110 Mary Foley's house in Connecticut; 113 ph Chris Everard/The London apartment of the Sheppard Day Design Partnership; 114 Kathy Moskal's apartment in New York designed by Ken Foreman; 115a The Sawmills Studios; 116–117 ph Andrew Wood/Phillip Low, New York; 117 ph Catherine Gratwicke; 118 ph David Montgomery; 121 Mary Foley's house in Connecticut.

# architects and designers

Work by the following architects and designers has been featured in this book:

Azman Associates
(formerly Azman Owens
Architects)
18 Charlotte Road
London EC2A 3PB
UK
tel: +44 (0)20 7739 8191
fax: +44 (0)20 7739 6191
Pages 28–29, 102–3.

behun/ziff design
153 E. 53rd Street
43rd Floor
New York, NY 10022
tel: 212 292 6233
fax: 212 292 6790
Page 63c.

Lisa Bynon Garden Design
P.O. Box 897
Sag Harbor, NY 11963
tel: 631 725 4680
Pages 106.

Ken Foreman
Architect
105 Duane Street
New York. NY 10007
tel/fax: 212 924 4503
Page 114.

Lulu Guinness
3 Ellis Street
London SW1X 9AL
UK
tel: +44 (0)20 7823 4828
fax:. +44 (0)20 7823 4889
www.luluguinness.com
Pages 73, 91.

John C Hope Architects
3 St Bernard's Crescent
Edinburgh EH4 1NR
UK
tel: +44 (0)131 315 2215
fax: +44 (0)131 315 2911
Page 6.

Mona Nerenberg
Home & garden products
and antiques
Bloom
43 Madison Street
Sag Harbor, NY 11963
tel: 631 725 4680
Page 106.

Jennifer Post Design
Spatial & Interior Designer
25 East 67th Street, 8D
New York NY 10021
tel: +1 212 734 7994
fax:. +1 212 396 2450
jpostdesign@aol.com
Page 100.

Lena Proudlock
www.lenaproudlock.com
Page 109.

Sheppard Day Design
tel: +44 (0)20 7821 2002
Page 113.

# index

**a**

acidophilus 46
affirmations 22–5
air-freshener 64
animal symbolism 116, 119
antioxidants 46
aromatherapy 64–5
   bath soak 55
   facial oil 56
assertiveness 91

**b**

bath oils 55, 64
beans 47
body detox 34–67
body language 79, 80
breastfeeding (caution) 41

**c**

candle meditation 59
children (caution) 64
cleansing ceremony 121
clothes 80–1
clutter-control 27, 102, 106–9
color 80–1
   in the home 115
cranberries 46
crystals 61

**d**

dairy products 44, 45
diabetes (caution) 41
diet 38–41
   culinary herbs and spices 46,
      47, 63
   foods to avoid 45
   superfoods 47
   two-week detox 44–6
   weekend detox 42–3

**e**

element symbolism 116
essential oils 64–5
   bath soak 55
   facial oil 56
exercise (physical) 48–9
   routine 50–1
exercises (self-improvement)
   candle-watching meditation
      59
   dissolving-barriers meditation
      424
   detoxing a friendship 88
   goal-setting 124
   harmony meditation 89

   tuning in to intuition 28
   letting-go meditation 31
   boosting self-respect 92
   visualization 23

**f**

face
   cleansing 55
   massaging 56–8
flirting tips 79
focus 27
   using role models 91
food 38–9, 41
   culinary herbs and spices
      46, 47, 63
   foods to avoid 45
   superfoods 47
   two-week detox 44–6
   weekend detox 42–3
friendship 83–9
fruit 46, 47

**g**

goal-setting 15–18
   using crystals 61
   daily 123–5
   for physical exercise 49
   using role models 91

**h**

habits
   bad 86
   good 27, 92
hair rinse 55
hay fever 41
headaches 46
herbs 62–3
   for detox diet 46, 47
home 96–121
      energy flow in 104–5, 118–19
      hidden meanings in 100–3
      mood-lifting 105
      protecting 119

**i**

image (appearance)
   of living space 100–3,
      110–17
   personal 78–81
inner critic 13, 74
intuition 27–9
irritable bowel syndrome 41

**j**

job interviews 91

**k**

kelp 46

**l**

legumes 47
letting go
   of negative feelings 89
   of relationships 84, 88
   of worries 30–1
linseed 46

**m**

massage 56–8
   oils 64
medical conditions
      (cautions) 41, 65
meditation 58
   candle watching 59
   for dissolving barriers
      24
   for harmony 89
   for letting go 31
milk thistle 46
mind detox 8–33

**n**

neatness 27
nuts 47

**o**

oats 46
oils
   culinary 47
   essential 55, 56, 64–5
organization 27

**p**

pampering 58
personality types 73–7
planning 14–19
plants 115
   symbolism of 117, 119
positive habits 27, 92
pregnancy (cautions) 41, 65
probiotics 46
problem-solving 88
protective symbolism 119

**q**

quinoa 46

**r**

relationship detox 68–95
rice 46
role models 91

**s**

seaweeds 47
seeds 46, 47
self-esteem 91–2
self-sabotage 25
self-talk 22–5
skin
   cleansing 55
   dry 64
   side effects 46
   sleep 52–3
space detox 96–121
   *see also* home
spices 47
stress-release 58
superfoods 47
supplements 46
symbolism
   of animals 116
   of natural elements 116
   of plants 117
   protective 119

**t**

thinking style 32, 33
time-management 18, 124
   time-wasters 27
toxic relationships 83–8, 91–2
toxic types 84
troubleshooting
   body 67
   home 121
   mind 33
   relationships 95
two-week detox 44–6

**v**

vegetables 46, 47
vision, personal 13
visualization 21–3, 25
   for dissolving barriers 24
   for letting go 31
   for harmony 89

**w**

water 40–1
   and exercise 49
   recommended daily
      intake 47
   symbolism 116
weekend detox diet 42–3
whole grains 46, 47
worries
   letting go of 30–1
   and sleep 53